Fifty & Fabulous

Fifty & Fabulous

Zia's Definitive Guide
to Anti-Aging—Naturally!

Zia Wesley-Hosford

with
Mary Earle Chase

Prima Publishing

PRIMA PUBLISHING and colophon are registered trademarks of Prima Communications, Inc.

Cover design by Lindy Dunlavey, The Dunlavey Studio
Cover photograph by Larry Dyer

Library of Congress Cataloging-in-Publication Data

Wesley-Hosford, Zia.
    Fifty & fabulous : Zia's definitive guide to anti-aging—naturally! / Zia Wesley-Hosford with Mary Earle Chase.
       p.   cm.
    Includes index.
    ISBN 1-55958-692-3
    ISBN 0-7615-0446-X (pbk.)
    1. Skin—Care and hygiene. 2. Aging. 3. Longevity.
I. Chase, Mary Earle. II. Title. III. Title: Fifty and fabulous.
RL87.W483 1995
646.7'26—dc20   94-39030
                                CIP

96 97 98 99 00 01 AA 10 9 8 7 6 5 4 3 2 1

Printed in the United States of America

How to Order

Single copies of this book may be ordered from Prima Publishing, P.O. Box 1260BK, Rocklin, CA 95677, telephone (916) 632-4400. Quantity discounts are also available. On your letterhead, include information concerning the intended use of the books and the num-ber of books you wish to purchase.

Visit us online at http://www.primapublishing.com

For my mother,
Ethel,
who has been fabulous
at every age.

Acknowledgments

Many thanks to all of the clients, friends, coworkers, family members, and guardian angels, who encouraged me to take "the next big step" in my life: to pursue my vision and create the company of my dreams, Educated Beauty.

Thank you to all the "human guinea pigs" who tried (and loved) all my new products, and to the thousands of readers whose continual feedback lets me know that I've helped make a difference in their lives.

A special thanks to my husband David for being my Rock of Gibraltar.

Contents

Fifty & Fabulous

Introduction

How many times have you heard someone "older" say, "If only I'd known then what I know now"? *Welcome to now.* I can't think of anything more exciting than approaching the second half of life with energy, intelligence, glowing health, and all the accumulated knowledge of the past 51 years! The possibilities are endless. Think of all you've learned in the past 40 or 50 years. Can you imagine learning just as much in the next 40? Even if you only learn half as much, it's going to be a great ride. I also believe learning has everything to do with staying young in mind, body, and spirit. Once the body, mind, or spirit become stagnant or inactive, we begin the decline commonly known as "aging" or "old age." I am not attempting to advocate immortality, but it is not inevitable that we become decrepit. I know many people in their seventies, eighties, and nineties who are fully aware, active, and functioning . . . many of whom still run their own businesses, write books, teach classes, have loving relationships, and travel the world. They are role models for successful living, and they share many similar character traits and habits, some of them so basic as to sound overly simplistic. In fact they are simple—easy to adapt and easy to incorporate into your life. This book tells you how to stay young in mind, body, and spirit.

Begin with the Skin

Only one body organ announces to the world how old or young you are—your skin. Think about it. The skin is the largest visible organ, covering an area of about 21 square feet on the average adult and weighing about nine pounds.

The skin is not just an inert wrapping; rather, it is very much alive and very busy, performing myriad duties vital to the life of the body. Functioning continuously, the skin protects the body from the invasion of bacteria, regulates the body's temperature, and takes in the oxygen that is necessary for the production of new cells, blood, and plasma. Millions of sensory nerve endings located throughout the skin give us our sense of touch and send warning signals to the brain and other organs. Twenty-four hours a day, the skin releases toxic waste through sweat glands and pores and manufactures sebum, the body's natural moisturizer. While we can replace some organs, such as the colon, kidneys, and heart, no one could live close to a normal life without skin.

Fortunately, the skin is very dependable and resilient. Just think of the countless cuts, burns, scrapes, and scratches you've endured and how efficiently your skin has healed itself. Regardless of how we may mistreat it, there is no such thing as "skin failure," and no one dies of "old skin."

Perhaps because the skin is so resilient, we tend to assume that it will take care of itself. To a point, it will. The skin continues to function as best it can, despite our abuse and neglect. As with other aspects of our lives, many of us don't start to care for our skin until it gives us trouble. We blithely go through our teens and twenties, taking our smooth skin for granted, maybe treating the occasional pimple. When we are young, the skin is very forgiving—it always seems to recover.

Then, usually after age 30, the signs of aging begin to appear. In general, fine lines around the eyes appear first; then the skin may become drier, rough, or discolored, and we may see more wrinkles and lines. Skin cancers, a direct result of sun exposure, begin to show up in one out of every three Americans over age 30. As we approach midlife, the cumulative damage of decades of neglect and abuse "suddenly" becomes apparent.

The sad fact is that most of these symptoms could have been avoided by a lifetime of care, beginning in childhood. *But regardless of what state your skin is in or how old you are, real improvements can be made.* While you may not be able to recapture your 20-year-old face, you can erase "years" of damage, naturally and nonsurgically. This book sets forth an anti-aging program that will help you achieve and maintain healthy, younger-looking skin. Skin problems of all kinds can be repaired with proper treatment, which includes working from the inside out with good nutrition, supplemental vitamins, and exercise; and working from the outside in with daily skin care, appropriate use of cosmetics, and various nonsurgical skin and body treatments.

My Own Path to Younger-Looking Skin

I am a prime example of someone who has used the information contained in this book to "take years off" my face. I initially became interested and involved in the cosmetics field 20 years ago when I attempted to solve some very serious skin problems of my own. At the time, I had been living for 8 years on the beach in Malibu, baking in the sun year-round and getting as dark a tan as possible. At age 30, my skin showed the typical "leathery" look of serious sun damage. It was lined, wrinkled, covered with red and brown blotches, and I was beginning to look older than my years.

At the same time, I developed a severe case of adult acne, which sent me on the rounds of dermatologists and estheticians, none of whom were able to help. I tried antibiotics (which resulted in dry skin, upset stomach, and yeast infections) and topical treatments that dried my skin out so thoroughly it was constantly peeling. I endured weekly ultraviolet light treatments followed by dry-ice "sloughing" at the dermatologists. (We now know that UV light ages the skin and causes cancer!) I tried dozens of different facialists and spent thousands of dollars, over a two-year period, on just about every brand name of cosmetics on the market. None offered a money-back guarantee, so I eventually threw away most of the products, many of which had only made my skin worse.

Finally, an esthetician at a salon in Beverly Hills introduced me to some European cosmetics made with botanicals (essential oils derived from plants) that actually brought improvement. She also encouraged me to investigate the link between skin problems and nutrition, which led me to consult nutritionists and herbalists, including two Native American healers. As I began to explore alternatives in herbal medicine, natural cosmetics, and diet and nutrition, my skin began to improve along with my health. I became so excited by the difference a holistic approach to skin care could make that I decided to pursue a career as a cosmetologist.

Four years later, after graduating from the Vidal Sassoon Academy in San Francisco, I opened a small salon in Sausalito and began to seek out high-quality products to use on my clients. I was shocked to find that such products did not exist. Taking a close look at cosmetics and their ingredients was like opening Pandora's box: Almost all of the products I evaluated—no matter where they were made—were of very low quality and sold at very high prices. I was enraged by what seemed to me a major consumer rip-off. Not only were the cosmetics of poor quality, they seemed to be responsible for many of the skin problems that plagued my clients.

I began to type up pages of information for my clients, warning them about specific products and ingredients to avoid. After two years, I had enough material for my first book, *Being Beautiful* (published by Whatever Publishing), which included the first layperson's cosmetic ingredient dictionary. To promote sales of my book at the American

Booksellers Association convention, I gave personal 10-minute consultations in my publisher's booth. One woman who came to see me had every skin problem you could imagine: acne, blackheads, dark circles under her eyes, excessive oiliness, large pores, sallowness, and premature aging. I explained that to make real improvements on her skin would take a change in lifestyle as well as cosmetics. She replied that she was tired of having bad skin and would try anything. So I recommended radical changes in her diet and her use of cosmetics, nutritional supplements, exercise, and that she quit smoking and—ideally—move to a less stressful living environment. Three weeks later she called me from New York, and I immediately remembered her. She said that she'd followed my instructions to the letter, and that she and her husband were even planning on moving out of the city. She said that in just three weeks her skin had changed radically and that she now had good skin for the first time in her life. "If you could do this for me," she said, "you can help thousands of others. I'm the senior editor of trade paperbacks at Bantam Books, and I'd like you to write a book for me." Bantam Books published my next book, *Putting On Your Face*. It sold over 200,000 copies and gained best-seller status, establishing me as the first cosmetics consumer advocate in the nation. Over the next three years, I wrote two more books for Bantam: *Face Value: Skin Care for Women Over 35* and *The Beautiful Body Book*.

During that time, I was also a skin-care instructor, working with about 40 students a week. I taught for a period of four years, and I was able to track my students' skin problems and to see what worked and didn't work to solve them. As I discovered patterns and developed solutions, I tried them on my clients—with remarkable results. Prescribing a holistic approach to all types of skin problems, I suggested changes in diet, introduced vitamins and exercise, and sought to reduce stress. I also recommended using cosmetics formulated from natural ingredients, but there were few quality products to be found. For this reason, I began mixing up my own cosmetics and sharing the "recipes" with my clients. These homemade natural products were the humble beginnings of Zia Cosmetics, and the forerunners of the state-of-the-art cosmetics I currently offer.

Over the past 14 years, I have met the challenge of wearing two hats: one as president of my own cosmetics company and one as a consumer advocate and author of eight books on skin care. Because I feel so strongly that consumers need objective advice about cosmetics and their ingredients, I work very hard to maintain my role as a skin-care educator and evaluator of skin-care products. Through my current company, Educated Beauty, Inc., I give people the most up-to-date, accurate information about solving skin problems and buying skin-care products. I still recommend products other than my own, regularly evaluating them via my online service. I also personally answer questions via e-mail. You may contact me at http://www.educatedbeauty.doc or Zia@educatedbeauty.com, or call my consumer line: 888-3ADVICE (323-8423).

The Proof Is in the Picture

Let's get back to my own skin and the results of all my efforts to repair the damage. *All I can say is that the proof is in the picture.*

The *before* picture of me (on the back cover) was taken in 1982 in bright natural light by Wernher Krutein. I was not wearing any foundation makeup or blush. I was 37 years old and had just recently stopped intentional tanning.

The *after* picture (on the back cover) was taken by Abhijit Varde in March 1994 after consistently eschewing tanning for 12 years. During that time, I had made changes in my diet, taken up aerobic exercise, and been on a program of nutritional supplements. In addition, for the past 10 years, I have used my own skin-care products, several of which I believe represent a breakthrough in cellular-renewal skin care. I used papaya enzyme on a daily basis for seven years, a natural alphahydroxy acid product for one year, and my poi and cranberry betahydroxy acid products for the past year. I believe my Vitamin A Elixir has helped to erase and soften expression lines even more while my natural anti-oxidant sunblock moisturizer absolutely prevents the occurrence of any new sun damage.

The before picture shows that my face is covered with brown spots, freckles, red spots, and broken capillaries. All of those discolorations are gone in the after photo. The texture of my skin in the before picture shows the beginning of a rough, leathery surface. Now, my skin is completely smooth. The aging lines on my face have also changed dramatically. The horizontal lines on my forehead are gone, and the laugh lines around my eyes are no more prominent, even though I have had 13 more years of smiling! The skin tone is as taut as it was 13 years earlier. Since the addition of my 5 Minute Cranberry Neck Cream, the skin on my neck has noticeably improved.

I am living proof that aging, sun-damaged, and problem skin can be treated effectively and that your skin can look younger as you grow older! I have written this book to share all that I know about how you too can slow and reverse the aging process. My philosophy combines my two decades of experience in the field of skin care with the wisdom I have received from teachers of all sorts—herbalists, acupuncturists, nutritionists, exercise instructors, and meditation teachers. They have all contributed to the holistic approach I believe is essential to having younger-looking skin as well as staying young in body, mind, and spirit.

If you want to look and feel better as you grow older, this book will tell you how.

1 Breakthroughs in Anti-Aging

One of the most exciting medical breakthroughs in the past decade has been the discovery of the skin's unsuspected properties and powers. As a result of new technologies employed in skin research over the past 15 years, we are experiencing what some have called a renaissance, both in the study of the skin as well as in the science of skin care. Simultaneously, a great deal of research is being done on the process of aging. As the baby boom generation approaches middle age, there is increased interest in what causes aging and how to prevent it.

Breakthroughs in these two areas of research have converged in discoveries of new products and treatments for aging skin as well as new attitudes about skin care. Some new products are hype and hoopla, but many of them actually do what they claim. Cosmetic companies have always promised that their products would make us look better and younger, and at last there is some validity to those claims!

The Epidermis: Alive and Interactive

The major breakthrough in skin science is an understanding of the epidermis, the outer layer of the skin that is very thin (no thicker than a piece of paper) and almost transparent. Until the late 1970s, scientists viewed the epidermis as a sheet of essentially dead cells that served as a protective barrier, sort of like a layer of Saran Wrap over the body. Then, in 1979, a team of researchers at the University of California at San Francisco discovered that the epidermis is a very permeable barrier, allowing many substances, depending on the size and structure of their molecules, to penetrate into the body. Now we know that *the epidermis is the primary pathway through the surface of the skin to the dermis, where many skin problems as well as aging occur.* By the early 1980s, new techniques in biochemistry and molecular biology led to the discovery that the epidermis is actually metabolically active and that it can stimulate responses within the body.

Another very significant discovery was that the epidermis plays a major role in providing immune protection, not just for the skin but for the entire body. Scientists found that the epidermis contains about half of the immune system's white blood cells, or leukocytes—cells that mobilize to fight viruses, bacteria, and cancer. This discovery seems to imply that the skin is responsible for almost half of the body's defense system. Other epidermal cells—melanocytes, keratinocytes, Langerhans cells, and Granstein cells—also play vital roles in the body's immune functions by producing various enzymes and hormones. Keratinocytes produce a hormone that enhances the growth of T cells, and they also synthesize a substance that stimulates immune-system response. It follows, then, that overall body health as well as how we age is directly related to skin health.

Epidermal cells help protect the body not only from invasion by bacteria and viruses, but also against damage from the sun. Nestled in the epidermis are melanocytes, the cells that give the skin its color. Melanocytes, which contain the pigment melanin, cause the skin to tan—a protection against the effects of the sun's ultraviolet rays.

The epidermis is made up of multiple layers of skin cells, with new cells being generated at the basal layer and traveling to the top layer, or *stratum cornum*. By the time they reach the *stratum cornum*, the cells are dead and are eventually sloughed off and replaced by underlying cells. This process of cellular renewal takes about 28 days— 14 days for the newborn cells to make it to the surface where they live for another 14 days. Epidermal renewal happens between midnight and 4:00 A.M., while other body systems are taking a rest. When first born, the new "epithelial" cells are round and filled with fluid. As they make their way up toward the surface of the skin, they lose their fluid, becoming elongated and flat. A water-resistant protein called keratin takes over the structure of the cell. These "keratinized" cells keep water from penetrating or evaporating from the body. After these cells reach the outer layer of the skin, they fall off during the process of washing or rubbing. As we get older, this shedding, or exfoliating, process slows down, causing a buildup of dead, dry cells—often most apparent on the lower legs.

Viewed under a microscope, epidermal cell structure seems to resemble a brick-and-mortar wall—protein cells stacked up and held together by what is called "intercellular cement." This cement, however, is not at all hard, but more like a gelatinous substance made up of lipids (fats) and waterlike fluids. This lipid network is the primary pathway for substances to enter the skin. The intercellular cement also seems to play a major role in skin appearance: When the fluids are in balance, the skin is "normal" (smooth and soft), but when there are imbalances in the lipid and water levels, the skin will look dry and feel rough and flaky. Skin researchers are now focusing on lipids in the search for answers to many skin problems, including aging.

These new discoveries about the epidermis mean that caring for that thin layer of surface skin may be more important than we ever imagined, so it's critical to understand the function of the epidermis and its relationship to the skin layer directly underneath, called the dermis.

Down in the Dermis

Beneath the epidermis lies the dermis, which is made up of collagen and elastin protein fibers woven together in a microscopic network like threads in fabric. This network forms the basic structure, or "skeleton," of the skin, similar to a mesh netting. Collagen gives the skin the ability to stretch, while elastin enables it to spring back into shape. Within the collagen and elastin fibers are the sweat glands, which control temperature and remove wastes, and the sebaceous glands, which manufacture and secrete sebum. This substance, so vital to the health and beauty of the skin, is actually a mixture of oil and water that is the skin's natural moisturizer. The dermis also includes the fat cells that insulate against cold, the network of capillary and lymph endings that bring in nutrients and eliminate toxins, and the nerve endings that carry sensations of pleasure or pain or the warning signs of danger to the rest of the body.

All of the processes that take place within the dermis depend on the healthy maintenance of the epidermis in order to function properly. For example, if the epidermis is clogged with a buildup of dead cells, sweat, and toxins, then excess sebum may become trapped beneath the skin, causing breakouts, whiteheads, and skin bumps. Hair follicles that become encrusted with a buildup of dry skin cause a condition called *keratosis pilaris,* which is characterized by tiny, hard bumps on the skin that appear most often on the upper arms and thighs.

Beneath the dermis is a bottom layer of subcutaneous fat that helps modulate body temperature and provides a cushion against trauma. All three—the epidermis, dermis, and fat—begin to thin out with age. Because the capillary network within them is reduced, there is less blood flowing to the skin. The results can be dryness, loss of elasticity, and changes in texture and color (those annoying "age spots"), as well as greater sensitivity. Older people often experience cold more acutely and bruise easier because of less insulation around their blood vessels.

But the most distressing signs of aging skin are the wrinkles and lines that appear on the face. And while to some of us those wrinkles might signify wisdom, most of us would just as soon never see them appear. Our new understanding of the role of the epidermis—its permeability, interactivity, and immune function—is shedding new light on wrinkles, and extensive research is being focused on the causes of facial lines and on developing products to help reduce or eliminate them.

The Wrinkles of Time

There are actually three kinds of wrinkles: expression, temporary, and aging lines. *Expression lines* are the result of facial expressions such as smiling, frowning, or squinting. They can show up as early as in our twenties, but usually become more and more pronounced the older we get. Facial expressions are the most benign cause of wrinkles because many of these "natural" or "character" lines give our faces the looks that make them individually our own. When they appear on a face that is healthy and well cared for, laugh lines around the eyes and smile lines around the mouth show that we feel and enjoy life. Few of us would choose to live a deadpan existence just to avoid these lines. Frown lines and the horizontal lines that can appear on the forehead, however, don't add character and are unnecessary. These lines can be avoided by not frowning or lifting your eyebrows continually in an expression of surprise. Expression lines already present can be minimized or even erased if you change your habits and stop making the expressions that cause them.

Temporary lines can also show up at an early age as a result of skin dehydration. These lines are very fine and usually appear on the cheeks. You can avoid them by using cosmetics that are appropriate for your skin type, protecting your face from the sun, and drinking lots of water. They can be treated very successfully with hydrating treatment products such as essential oils, masks, and moisturizers, along with exfoliating products.

Aging lines are the deeper wrinkles we are all most concerned with. Fine lines appear around the eyes and deep lines may appear on the forehead, cheeks, neck, and chest as the skin begins to sag. In the past decade, we have come to understand more about why aging lines occur and how they can be prevented or minimized.

As we've seen, our epidermal cells are constantly renewing themselves—in our youth, about every 30 days. But as we age, that renewal process takes longer and longer to produce fresh skin, and by our sixties, the cycle can take as long as 60 days. We don't really know why this slowdown takes place, but we do know that during this longer time span, a lot more can go wrong with skin cells. Epidermal cells pile up and become progressively dehydrated, resulting in rough, scaly skin.

Another factor in skin wrinkling is the breakdown of collagen and elastin. When collagen, the skin's major support structure, degenerates, the skin begins to sag. As the elastin fibers become stretched, tangled, and fragmented, the skin loses its ability to spring back into shape. These changes in collagen and elastin plus the mechanical forces of facial expressions, frowning and smiling or repetitive movements like pursing the lips, will eventually lead to wrinkles or lines.

The Role of Free Radicals in Aging

One theory about why the collagen and elastin fibers begin to break down with age concerns the activities of "free radicals." No, the term doesn't refer to the political activists of the 1960s, but to certain oxygen molecules believed to be responsible for damaging other cells and causing aging and disease. Only in the past decade have we come to understand the role of free radicals and how they operate in the body.

Free radicals are the by-products of the burning of oxygen (oxidation) in our cells; therefore, free radicals are crucial to life itself. But when they proliferate, they "feed on" other cells. Because free radicals are unstable oxygen molecules, lacking an electron, they attack other molecules and steal their electrons, leaving those molecules out of balance. Free radicals attack DNA and RNA, the lipids in cellular membranes, and the proteins in collagen and elastin. It is this damage to the skin cells that causes wrinkled, sagging, discolored skin.

There are many factors that increase free-radical production. The primary one is bombardment of the skin by the sun's ultraviolet rays. Other factors include pollutants that affect the skin either internally or externally. The breathing in of cigarette smoke or smog; the consumption of alcohol, drugs, or toxic substances in food; and exposure to chemicals in substances we come in contact with—all of these factors put our skin under siege. We'll be looking more closely at free-radical producers in Chapter 3.

Combating the proliferation of free radicals is the body's aggressive protective system of antioxidants. The antioxidants are an army of chemicals that seek out free radicals to which they attach themselves in order to prevent their attack on other cells. The antioxidants thereby neutralize and detoxify the free radicals, which are then flushed from the body. Antioxidant substances include vitamins A, C, E, and beta-carotene, as well as various trace minerals and enzymes. I'll talk more about these anti-aging supplements in Chapter 5.

Wrinkling of the facial skin, then, is the result of a combination of factors—the slowing down of epidermal renewal and the breaking down of collagen and elastin when under attack by free radicals. Cellular renewal is the process of repairing and healing the skin by increasing the rate of cell production. The new skin-care products designed to rid the skin of wrinkles can be classified as cellular-renewal products. Retinoic acid, alphahydroxy acids, enzyme peels, liposomes, oxygenation, and topically applied vitamins are all aimed at speeding up cell renewal and boosting collagen production.

Let's take a look at these products and the all-important question, Do they work?

Retin-A: Antiwrinkle Miracle?

There has been a great deal of excitement about the wrinkle-reducing properties of Retin-A, a prescription drug used for many years to treat acne. With much fanfare, it was announced in 1988 that studies had shown Retin-A to have positive effects on aging skin, erasing superficial lines and wrinkles, improving skin texture, and evening out skin tone. Immediately, people without acne got their doctors to prescribe the drug, and Retin-A sales skyrocketed. The hope (and the hype) was that Retin-A would be a miracle drug for wrinkled skin, allowing us all to return to the smooth skin of yesteryear. In the past few years, however, the drug has lost most of its reputation as a fountain of youth.

Retin-A is the brand name of a vitamin-A derivative also known as retinoic acid and tretinoin, and no one is quite sure yet how it works on the skin. It seems to stimulate the rate of cell turnover in the epidermis, so that new cells replace dead ones at a faster rate. It may also speed up the production of collagen and elastin and increase blood flow to the epidermis. Whatever it does, Retin-A does seem to "plump up" the skin and thicken the epidermis, thus making wrinkles less apparent. The results take place over a period of three months to a year and seem to last only as long as Retin-A continues to be used.

The main problem with Retin-A is that it has several negative side effects. It irritates the skin, making it sensitive to many skin-care products as well as to the sun. In fact, while using Retin-A, you must wear a sunblock with a minimum SPF (sun protection factor) of 15, daily, to avoid sunburn and the development of dark pigmentation. If you are caught in the sun unprotected, the skin will burn within a matter of minutes. While using Retin-A, the skin becomes very red and will also peel and flake for several months. Many people who used it also felt their skin became sensitive to the touch. Those with very fair skin may not be able to use Retin-A at all because of its harsh side effects.

Many researchers are doubtful whether Retin-A is the miracle antiwrinkle drug it claims to be. They question whether the effects of the drug are simply the same as the effects of any substance that "gooses" the skin, causing mild irritation and inflammation—another form of skin plumping. No one knows what the long-term effects of using this product will be, and there is speculation that it may affect the DNA of skin cells. Scientists do seem to agree that the effects of retinoic acid need a great deal more study.

My own experience is that Retin-A users have been uniformly disappointed with the results. In dozens of skin seminars, I have asked hundreds of people how many have tried using Retin-A to reduce wrinkles. Usually, about a third of each audience will raise their hands. When I ask how many are still using it, no hands go up. Most people complain of the substantial side effects that prevent continued usage.

The jury is still out on Retin-A, but if you would like to try it, you should get a prescription from a dermatologist who knows about the side effects and who can instruct you on how to use it properly. She or he should then monitor the results with follow-up visits to make sure that your skin is responding favorably.

The FDA has approved an over-the-counter version of Retin-A called Renova, which will soon come on the market as a topical cream to treat "premature aging." I don't know what difference there is between Renova and Retin-A, or whether Renova will have the same irritating side effects. Even if it does not, it will be important to consider the ingredients that are included along with the retinoic acid. Look to see if the formulation contains mineral oil, chemicals, or fragrance. If so, you may not want to put it on your skin, especially since there are natural alternatives that work just as well—alphahydroxy acids and enzyme peels—without the negative side effects.

Alternatives to Retin-A

Alphahydroxy and Betahydroxy Acids

The best news in treating aging skin is not a chemical concoction, but rather some natural, nontoxic acids that are proving to be as effective as Retin-A and yet easier on the skin and on the pocketbook. These acids are commonly referred to as fruit acids.

Alpha and Betahydroxy acids are a gentle, effective, and less expensive way to treat wrinkles and a variety of other skin problems. Both acids remove dead skin cells in two ways: first, by loosening the intercellular cement between the old and new epidermal cells; second, by very efficiently dissolving the dead surface cells. This gentle exfoliation process means that younger cells are more visible on the surface of the skin. Thus, these gentle acids soften fine lines and wrinkles, making them less visible. With fewer dead cells on the surface of the skin, skin texture improves and discolored patches begin to disappear. They benefit both oily and dry skin by removing the dead cells that clog pores and cause breakouts in oily skin, or that get in the way of moisturization in dry skin. There is evidence that fruit acids also help to get rid of wrinkles by boosting collagen production. When used on a regular basis, over time, they help rid the skin of brown spots and precancerous conditions.

There are many forms of fruit acids, including glycolic acid from sugarcane; malic acid from apples; citric acid from oranges, lemons, and limes; tartaric acid from wine grapes; and lactic acid from milk and salysylic from white willow bark and meadowsweet. These various acids work in different ways: glycolic acid from sugarcane has the smallest molecules and therefore penetrates deeper and faster; lactic acid has larger molecules and stays on the surface to help the sloughing-off of the uppermost cells.

In very high concentrations—solutions of 30 to 70 percent fruit acid—AHAs are used by dermatologists and plastic surgeons for facial peels. The process burns away the top layer of the skin and thus reduces fine lines and wrinkles. Because these peels are very strong and can result in problems, they must be applied by a qualified physician. I will discuss this type of peel in Chapter 7. Prescription-strength AHA creams, with 12 to 20 percent fruit acid, are used to treat skin problems such as ichthyosis—severely dry, scaly skin.

We are currently seeing a boom in over-the-counter AHA and BHA products designed for daily skin-care use. Almost every cosmetics company now has some type of alphahydroxy-acid formulation, all using different fruit acids and different concentrations, from 1 to 12 percent. Almost all of these products employ the chemical forms of glycolic acid or lactic acid that, unfortunately, can make them difficult to use on a daily basis.

The concentration of AHAs in a skin-care product is important, as most people cannot tolerate more than a 4 to 6 percent concentration on a daily basis. Redness, itching, and breakouts are the most common complaints. Some of these symptoms are caused by the acids themselves and some are caused by buffers. When the chemical form of an AHA is used in a product, a buffering agent must be used as well, and the buffers themselves are irritating. One commonly used buffering agent is sodium hydroxide, or lye, a caustic agent used to make soap. Another is triethanolamine (TEA), a commonly used cosmetic ingredient that is benign when used as less than 5 percent of a formulation; however, when TEA is used to buffer or balance an acid, it becomes a primary ingredient.

The FDA does not require companies to list percentages of AHA concentration, so it's difficult to know what you are getting. Companies that initially marketed high concentrations have had to reformulate them because people found them too irritating.

I choose to use only all natural, chemical-free sources of betahydroxy acids in my Provenance products which are gentle enough for everyday use by all skin types.

The effectiveness, then, of these products depends very much on the formulation of the ingredients. In proper formulation, they work as well if not better than Retin-A, and without the irritation and sun sensitivity. If you use an appropriate AHA or BHA product nightly, you will see results in two weeks to a month. Your skin will be smoother, lines will diminish, and you will have a more healthy looking "glow." Prolonged usage brings continual improvement. After 6 to 12 months, the skin texture, tone, and coloration may be restored to reflect little or no visible sun damage. This means no more redness, broken capillaries, brown spots, surface dehydration, slackness, or "crepeyness." In short, the result of appropriate use of fruit acids is smoother, moister, younger-looking skin. I think this rival to Retin-A truly is an antiwrinkle miracle worker!

Enzyme Exfoliants

Another stronger exfoliation process is accomplished by use of enzymes that digest the protein in dead skin cells and helps increase circulation, bringing nutrients and oxygen to the skin. Enzyme products may be composed of a variety of naturally occurring enzymes: papain from papayas, bromelain from pineapples, and—less commonly—enzymes from vegetable sources. Salons use enzyme peels exclusively for exfoliation. When used at home on a daily basis, they are an excellent cellular renewal treatment for healing sun damage, age spots, scarring, uneven skin coloration, and acne.

PrimeZyme Green Papaya Puree Mask is a natural alternative to Retin-A, made from organically grown green papayas, citrus fruit, raw Hawaiian honey, sunflower oil, and vitamin E. The active ingredient, papain, is a "proteolytic" enzyme, meaning it has the ability to selectively digest dead protein by dissolving the old cells without harming the younger, living cells. Papain has been used as a meat tenderizer and is also taken internally as a digestive aid. Powdered papaya has been added to some skin-care products for its exfoliating effect, but because ripe papaya was used to make the powder, it has little or no effect on the skin.

In order to be an effective exfoliant, the papain enzyme must be extracted from papayas that are young and green. Once the papaya begins to ripen and develop sugar, the enzyme activity decreases rapidly. Heat also destroys the enzyme, so it is important that the product be processed at a low temperature. Since a fresh green papaya product cannot be stored for long periods, it must be produced and shipped on a timely basis. Obviously, this is not a product that lends itself to mass production. This is why the Fresh Papaya Enzyme Peel is so unique.

The papaya enzyme product takes the place of traditional granular scrub exfoliants that can damage the skin by breaking capillaries. Because it doesn't activate oil glands like an abrasive, the enzyme product may be used by all skin types, including people with oily or combination skin. The best reason to choose an enzyme product over a grainy exfoliant is not just because of the enzyme but also because of the vitamins surrounding it. Vitamins A, C, and E are the most effective free-radical scavengers. The combined activity of the vitamins and the proteolytic enzyme helps boost the production of new collagen and elastin fibers for smoother, younger skin.

If you choose to use Retin-A, an enzyme peel can increase the effectiveness of the treatment as well as help alleviate the redness, flaking, and peeling that often occur.

The peel should be used in the morning, applied to the face and left on for 20 minutes, during which time it will digest the dead skin cells that have been brought to the surface during the night by Retin-A. I have found, however, that using the enzyme peel by itself will, over time, give the same results as the Retin-A, without any of the adverse side effects or sun sensitivity.

If you suffer from psoriasis or eczema, use the papaya peel several times a week to eliminate flaking skin anywhere on your body.

New Delivery System: Liposomes

In addition to generating new ingredients for skin-care products, recent breakthroughs in skin science have also identified new ways to deliver those ingredients into the skin. In many cases, to be most effective, a product must find its way to a precise location and remain there for a prescribed period of time. Enter the new delivery vessels, liposomes.

Liposomes are microscopic spheres composed of phospholipids (fats), which are a natural component of skin-cell membranes. Because a liposome's membrane is so similar to the outer membrane of skin cells, it is able to penetrate the cellular walls and deliver its contents deeper into the epidermis than other topically applied substances. Liposomes might be said to slip into the "empty spaces" in the skin caused by dehydration and free-radical damage. Once there, they "melt" and release their contents of lipids slowly over a period of about 10 to 12 hours.

Some cosmetic substances that previously could not be absorbed into the skin can now be absorbed with the help of liposomes. Moisturizing ingredients transported by liposomes are able to penetrate the skin more effectively than other moisturizers. As a result, liposomes are now being used in a variety of skin-care preparations including moisturizers, aftershaves, cleansing lotions, sunscreens, and tanning agents.

Most liposomes are made of lecithin, which is derived from egg yolk. Lecithin is a well-known phospholipid with a great ability to attract and hold water. Clinical studies have shown that liposomes promote natural moisturizing of the skin by reducing water loss. Depending on their composition, they also aid in repairing cellular damage and stimulating cellular turnover.

"The Latest": Oxygenation and Vitamins

Every month, it seems, the fashion magazines announce a "new breakthrough" in skin care, with quotes from the heads of research and development of all the major cosmetic companies about how their new line of products will "revolutionize" skin care. Some of the latest developments in cosmetics involve adding oxygen, vitamins, or provitamins to skin products.

One of the newest product developments is lacing moisturizers with oxygen to deliver this essential element directly to the cells. Proponents believe that oxygenation can actually breathe new life into old skin. You know the way your skin seems to glow after exercising? This is the result of oxygenation, in which oxygen travels through the bloodstream to the skin. The theory behind oxygenating moisturizers is this: As skin ages, cell walls thicken and capillary circulation decreases, making the absorption of oxygen more difficult. This, in turn, leads to "fatigued" skin cells that ultimately cause fine lines and wrinkles. Delivering oxygen topically is supposed to remedy this situation.

But wait a minute, you say, didn't I just read about oxidation causing the proliferation of those nasty free radicals? Yes, but keep in mind that oxygenation and oxidation are not the same process. Oxidation is the process of burning oxygen that takes place in the cells, producing by-products like free radicals, whereas oxygenation contributes oxygen to the cell. A few oxygenating products claim to contain antioxidants that counteract free-radical damage.

Some skin experts are skeptical about oxygenation products. While acknowledging that the amount of oxygen supplied to the skin decreases with age, they say that the ramifications of this have yet to be fully studied. Some say if you want to oxygenate the skin, just exercise or get a massage!

New oxygenated products are currently being introduced at quite a clip. Hydrogen peroxide is a popular ingredient currently being used to create oxygenation. Aloe vera is one of the oldest oxygenators available because it enables the skin to attract and hold oxygen, which in turn helps it to hold moisture. Since aloe vera has been used for thousands of years, I can't say that it represents a "breakthrough" skin-care product; it does, however, have cellular-renewal and antioxidant properties, which I discuss at length in Chapter 5. Another oxygenating product I have tested is Dermalive, which has been used with excellent results to treat psoriasis and eczema.

Many of the "latest" skin-care remedies coming on the market from the mass-market companies are cosmetics and makeup products that contain vitamins. It is curious that the fashion magazines consider this something new, since natural skin-care products have long contained vitamins A, E, C, and D. There is considerable evidence that the topical application of these vitamins promotes healing and helps to improve a wide variety of skin conditions, problems, and damage.

One truly new development is the use of provitamins, which are chemical precursors of the vitamins themselves, synthetically manufactured. We have been hearing about provitamin D-3, which is supposed to improve skin firmness

recommendations. To get answers to your personal skin-care questions or inquire about products you find in the marketplace, you can also e-mail me at Zia@educatedbeauty.com or call my toll-free number, 888-3ADVICE (323-8423).

2 The Mind–Body Connection and the Process of "Youthing"

At the time of this writing, Dr. Deepak Chopra's book *Ageless Body, Timeless Mind* has been a fixture on the *New York Times* Best-seller List for 36 weeks. What I find interesting is that Dr. Chopra isn't saying much that is new about aging. Basically, his recommendations for longevity include eating a healthy diet, getting moderate exercise, meditating daily, and changing one's attitudes and beliefs about aging. What is significant about his approach, however, is that it is finally reaching mainstream America.

For many years, I have been addressing aging from the point of view of "mind and body"—that is, that a person's belief system about aging may be the major factor in how that person's body ages. The following excerpt is taken from *The Beautiful Body Book: A Lifetime Guide for Healthy, Younger-Looking Skin*, which I wrote in 1988. This material appeared in Chapter 1, "Do Our Minds Control Our Bodies?"

In recent years, research has proven the amount of power that the mind exerts over the body. Various scientific experiments—auto suggestion, hypnosis, or biofeedback techniques—have had successful results in areas such as training people to steady their uneven heart rates, reducing high blood pressure, and improving hearing.

In a 1970 study in New Delhi, India, yoga practitioner Ramanand Yogi demonstrated the ability to slow his heart rate at will, decrease his intake of oxygen to one-fourth of the minimum required for the maintenance of human life, and cause perspiration to appear at an isolated point on his body (the forehead). Modern psychology now accepts the fact that a person's mental state affects and often controls the physical state. If this is so, how may our individual minds be programming our bodies?

Dr. Robert Morgan, dean for academic and professional affairs at the California School of Professional Psychology, and president of the Division of Gerontological Psychology for the International Association of Applied Psychology, regards the mind as a "dimension of the body rooted in the nervous system, not as something separate from the body. It is therefore important to the complete study of aging." Dr. Morgan defines aging as "a series of disadvantaging events that normally occur in our bodies over time. These events gradually reduce our ability to adapt to our surroundings in such a way that they increase the probability of death. The less efficient our bodies become, the more chances we have of dying." We may add years to our life spans by reducing the number of disadvantaging events in our lives.

For example, let's look at a factor that may very well be the number-one cause of aging: our belief systems— specifically the one about how old we're getting. From early childhood, we are exposed to the belief systems of those around us, and because of our naïveté, we are easily impressed by the beliefs that are held by older people whom we love and admire. As we grow up, these subliminally held beliefs begin to program us, just as they programmed our elders.

I've designed a short quiz to give you some concrete examples of how this works. It may also help you to discover your subconscious beliefs on the subject of aging. Read the statements through once, and see if you can

associate them with specific elders from your childhood.
Then reread them, and check the ones that you've found
yourself saying or thinking.

1. I guess I must be getting old.
2. That's just part of getting old.
3. I'm not getting any younger.
4. It's all downhill from here.
5. When I was young . . .
6. I'm not as young as I used to be.
7. When you're as old as I am . . .
8. Ever since I turned . . .

Reprogramming for Extended Youth

By the continued repetition of these and other lita-
nies, are we actually programming ourselves to age? I
believe that we are. Many teachers, researchers, and ther-
apists hold similar beliefs. Gerontologist Lawrence Casler
refers to statements such as those listed above as "self-
fulfilling prophecies." In an experiment with 30 residents
of The Jewish Home and Hospital for the Aged in New
York City, he proved that these beliefs could be successfully manipulated.

The 30 people were divided into two groups.
Members of the experimental group were visited by
Mr. Casler on a regular basis and given positive suggestions—sometimes by hypnosis, sometimes just by conversation—regarding their health and vitality. The suggestions went something like this: "A person is as young
as he feels . . . You may have many happy, healthy years
ahead of you—years full of opportunity for pursuing your
interests and hobbies and developing new ones, making
new friends and enjoying life free of financial and other
responsibilities . . . You will find it easy to relax, to enjoy
yourself, and to remain healthy and happy for many years

to come." Members of the control group received no visits or suggestions of any kind from Mr. Casler, but were left to their normal, everyday routine.

Mr. Casler followed up on his experimental and control groups one year after the sessions had ended and found that the experimental group had less sickness and fewer injuries and hospitalizations than the control group. Their rate of recovery was also markedly faster. Of the control group, 6 of the original 15 had died within the year, while only 1 of the experimental group had died. In the years that followed, the experimental group lived more than four times as long as the control group.

Using a slightly different technique, Leonard Elkind, a clinical psychologist and hypnotherapist in San Francisco, illustrated the impact of hypnosis on aging. He developed tests designed to measure the various effects of aging on different parts of the body. In these experiments, he used women between the ages of 39 and 53 and implanted positive thoughts regarding youth and vitality. Within four weeks, one session had reduced the subjects' "body age" (as measured by his methods of testing) by an average of 11 years.

Mr. Elkind describes hypnosis as a "technique that speaks to the part of the mind that regulates the body" and believes it to be the most powerful tool capable of intervening in the aging process. This does not mean that you need to begin extensive hypnotherapy treatment. In fact, Mr. Elkind states that all hypnosis is self-hypnosis and the therapist merely "helps to put his subject into a better hypnotic state." There are other practitioners who share similar beliefs and who have developed various types of self-help treatments based on theories such as these.

If you are under age 30, you're at an even greater advantage because you haven't yet reached the point of thinking of yourself as old. I believe that, with regard to age, you are as old or as young as you feel; the choice is yours. I now ask you to stretch your imagination a bit and play a little game with yourself. Pretend that it is possible to turn back the clock. Consciously make a decision to stop saying and thinking aging phrases and replace them with positive statements, such as "I feel great at [whatever age you are]" or "Life keeps getting better." Notice any changes in your mental attitude after just a week or so of this. If you see even a small improvement, take it one step further and decide what you'd like to change or improve about your body. Try some of the practices and suggestions in this book, and don't give up in a week or two. Remember that it took years for your skin and body to develop the signs of age that you notice, and it will take time to reverse the aging process. Many of the treatments I recommend begin to take effect after a period of one to three months. It may take two to three years for you to see the end results of the improvements you've envisioned. Program yourself for success, and give whatever you choose to try a realistic chance to work. Track your progress on a weekly or bimonthly basis, rather than daily. I'm currently working on a two- to three-year program to improve the sun-damaged skin on my body. The thought of looking younger in coming years is very appealing to me. After all, the years are going to go by anyway. Why not make them work *for* you?

Then and Now

It's interesting for me to read that passage, which I wrote almost ten years ago, at age 41. By the time you read this I will have already celebrated my fifty-first birthday. I still look and feel 15 years younger than my chronological age, and the past 10 years have more than ever boosted my belief in "mind over body." When I tell people my age, they invariably ask what my secret is. Without having to think, I always reply, "I'm too stubborn to get old." Actually, there is more truth in that than you may think. I have no concept of "old." I have no pictures in my mind about aging. Very simply, I don't see myself getting old. I see myself as young and vital. Life fascinates and excites me. I can't imagine being bored. My only problem seems to be able to fit into my day, week, month, and year, all of the things I want to do; there never seems to be enough time to get everything done, including doing nothing.

Recently, there has been some incredibly exciting research in the area of mind–body connection carried out by Dr. Candace Pert, professor of physiology and biophysics at Georgetown University. Dr. Pert's work, miles ahead of the rest of the field, is primarily concerned with neuropeptides (peptides for short), miniscule proteins produced by nerve cells that communicate messages from the brain to all organs of the body through the use of chemicals. The specifics of this communication verify the suspected link between emotions and the physical symptoms that signal disease. Simply put, your mind can make you sick. If this is true, reasons Dr. Pert, the reverse is also true: Your mind can make you well.

At 48 years old, Dr. Pert has been doing research on peptides for almost 25 years, at such respected institutions as Johns Hopkins Medical Center, Rutgers University, and the National Institutes of Health. Ten years ago, Dr. Pert went public with her opinion that peptides and their corresponding neuroreceptors, which occur throughout the body, are in fact a "psychosomatic" network run by our emotions. She believes that one day we may be able to influence our emotions as well as our physical status by using our mind to alter the "peptide cocktails"—mixtures of peptides continually produced by the body that signal the body's organs.

When I asked Dr. Pert how she felt her research with peptides might affect longevity, she initially replied, "That's an interesting question," and thought carefully for a moment before answering.

"A lot of what we think of as great medical care isn't. Mainstream medicine ignores the mind, except for psychiatry, which only considers the abnormal mind. So, I think the opportunity we have is to explore alternatives that place the mind in a more central position. There are so many other ways to feel better than to have your body operated on." This answer prompted me to ask how her research had impacted her life on a personal level. Her response didn't surprise me at all. "Let me just say," she replied, "that I've embraced many forms of consciousness training, which has helped me enormously."

Currently, the National Institutes of Health's newly established Office of Alternative Medicine is funding several studies to examine the effectiveness of alternative healing practices, including traditional Chinese medicine, acupuncture, biofeedback, t'ai chi ch'uan, transcendental meditation, and homeopathy. There are over 40 other NIH-funded studies on spirituality and religion, as these relate to health care. Other venerable institutions such as the Institute on Aging, the National Cancer Institute, and the Mental Health Institute are all involved in research to uncover the connection between good health and spirituality; the only group that seems to be missing from this impressive list is the American Medical Association. However, I know of hundreds of American physicians who have incorporated one or more forms of alternative medicine into their practices.

I strongly suspect that in the next decade we're going to discover that the mind has even more control over the body than we currently believe. For now, I can suggest some readily available tools that you can use, such as meditation, self-hypnosis, positive thinking, affirmations, creative visualizations (including the following one), and visioning. But regardless of which methods you choose, remember that the key lies in *your mind*. Use it well.

"Youthing" Through Visualization Meditation

I had my first experience with visualization when I was 12 years old. At the time, no one called it visualization. I had

7. Tell yourself, "My body becomes more relaxed every time I exhale." Do this for a minute or two.

8. Now begin a mental inventory of your body to ensure relaxation. Begin with picturing your feet and telling yourself, "My feet are relaxed." Continue with legs, hips, chest, arms, hands, neck, and face.

Visualizing the "Youthing" Process

After you have become accomplished with the above process, relaxing your mind and body, you can add the following visualization process.

1. In your mind, picture a big, bright, white light in the sky about 25 feet above the roof of the house or apartment you are in.

2. Imagine that the light emanating from this source creates a cone of light that encompasses the house in a huge circle.

3. When that light touches the ground, it becomes a pale purple, or amethyst, color and takes the form of cool flames circling the house. The flames move inward toward the center of the circle, up through the house, and into your body through the soles of your feet.

4. As the cool, amethyst-colored flames move through your body, see them "burn away" toxins, pain, negative emotions, and anything else you want to rid your body of. For example, if you have a pain in your knees, focus the healing ability of the flames there and picture them burning the pain away. (Always picture the flames as cool.)

5. Imagine the cool flames burning away the signs of aging in various areas of your body. See them "eating up" free radicals like Pac-Man, and see the problems you are concerned with turning to ashes and floating away. You can take as long as you like with this part of the process. When you are done, continue with the next step.

6. Imagine the flames carrying with them any negativity as they exit your body through a hole in the top of your head. See the negativity dissolving and disappearing into the air.

7. Picture the flames surrounding your body in an amethyst "cocoon," encircling you and protecting you.

8. Tell yourself that on the count of three you are going to open your eyes and feel either refreshed and full of energy or relaxed and ready to go to sleep.

This process may seem somewhat strange to you if you have never had any experience with visualization, but I assure you that it is very, very powerful. I have included it because it has been a very useful tool for me to use over the years, for healing as well as for "youthing." I encourage you to work on looking and feeling younger not only by what you do with your body but also by what you do with your mind.

Life is a process, the tiny steps we take along our path of moments, days, and years. Our end results, goals, and dreams help to give meaning and a sense of completion to the process of life. But sometimes we mistake our goals for life itself, when getting there is really what we need to pay attention to and to enjoy.

I encourage you to begin to pay attention to each moment of the process of your life and move toward your goals of health and beauty with enjoyment, challenge, and interest.

3

How and Why Skin Ages

The brave new world of skin science and skin-changing products is bringing hope to people whose skin is showing the ravages of age and to those who want to prevent damage before it occurs. We now have a better understanding of the structure and function of the skin and the processes that bring about its aging—the slowing of cell renewal and the breakdown of collagen and elastin because of free radicals. The good news is that skin damage is both reversible and preventable. The bad news is that if you want to keep your skin looking young, you are going to have to protect it meticulously from the sun.

Skin Enemy Number One: The Sun

Ultraviolet and infrared radiation from the sun are the major causes of aging skin. In fact, about 80 percent of what we consider skin aging symptoms are attributable to sunlight. If we were raised indoors and never exposed to sunlight, our skin would look very much the same at age 50 as it did at age 20. If you doubt this statement, examine the skin under your breasts and underarms and on your buttocks and compare that skin to the back of your hand. The only difference is the amount of sun exposure these areas receive. As you grow older, the skin not exposed to ultraviolet light will remain essentially unchanged. Unprotected areas such as the hands, face, and neck will develop lines and wrinkles, lose their elasticity, and change in texture and color.

These skin changes occur as a result of *incidental* exposure to the sun—walking outside, driving, playing sports, gardening, and such. A person who sunbathes *intentionally* will develop the tough, leathery skin and deeper expression lines and wrinkles that is often called "elephant skin." Picture an older women who has spent years of winters in Florida. In her youth, she may have been described as being "brown as a berry." Past the age of 45 or 50, she may be compared to a walnut.

The damage inflicted by the sun is called "photoaging." What happens is that the normal breakdown of collagen and elastin is accelerated by ultraviolet radiation. Skin cells that have been photodamaged also produce "deviant" types of collagen and elastin. Sunlight damage to keratinocytes and melanocytes can reduce the effectiveness of the immune system.

Individual photoaging is dependent on the amounts of two substances contained in the skin: (1) melanin, the body's natural sun-shielding substance that gives the skin its color; and (2) protective oil. The more melanin and oil, the thicker the skin is and the less likely it is to be damaged by the sun. The lighter and thinner the skin, the more prone it is to dry out, burn, and eventually wrinkle. As we know, people of Irish/English descent and redheads are generally more sun sensitive. Ancestry is one of the reasons why Australians are so susceptible to skin cancer: most originally emigrated from England. The darker and thicker the skin, the stronger it is and the less likely it is to show photoaging. Dark skin also tends to be oilier, so it doesn't dry out as early as light skin. All other factors being equal, fair-skinned people will often look older than their darker-skinned counterparts.

One of the worst aspects of sun damage is that it is cumulative. A person may tan for the first 25 years of her life without noticing any skin changes. The outward signs don't show up until after the damage has already been done. The best analogy I've heard was given on national television by a dermatologist who likened sun-tanning to the boiling of an egg. A whole raw egg may be submerged in boiling water for a few seconds with no apparent change. Submerge it for a few more seconds, and there is still no change. But if you continue to submerge it, for a few seconds at a time, at some point it will become hard-boiled.

Skin Cancer: The New Epidemic

If the prospect of dry, wrinkled, sagging skin isn't enough to scare you out of the sun, consider the serious, sometimes fatal, consequences of too much sun: skin cancer. According to the Skin Cancer Foundation, "The ultraviolet rays of the sun, in fact, are the most frequent cause of skin cancer. Deliberate, repeated sun-tanning and especially sunburns, increase the incidence of skin cancer. Sun exposure has a cumulative effect. Even though a suntan may disappear, the signs of skin cancer can show up years later." While intermittent exposure on a daily basis is most commonly linked to nonmalignant types of skin cancer, malignant melanomas are thought to be caused by intermittent doses of strong sun. The "vacation tan" that many people get once or twice a year can be the most dangerous.

In the past five decades, there has been a phenomenal increase in all types of skin cancers, and, while most are not life-threatening, the rate of malignant melanoma, the deadliest form, has soared. According to the American Academy of Dermatology, in 1935 only 1 out of every 1500 Americans could expect to develop malignant melanoma, but by 1985 the odds changed to 1 in 150. By the year 2000, the odds will be 1 in 100.

The American Academy of Dermatology also estimated that, in 1993, 32,000 people were diagnosed with melanoma and that 6800 people died from the disease. The causes of this type of often-fatal cancer are varied; until recently, researchers cited genetic elements, excessive exposure to ultraviolet light, intermittent doses of strong sun, immunological factors, and viral and chemical carcinogens as the causes. Although genetic inheritance can create a predisposition to melanoma, this type of skin cancer most often affects those who experienced damaging or repeated sunburns as teenagers. The newest research suggests that ultraviolet light suppresses the skin's immune system, which in turn hinders its ability to fight off the formation of melanomas. This would explain the test results published by the M. D. Anderson Cancer Center in Houston, Texas, which showed that sunscreens protected mice against sunburns and superficial skin cancers but not against melanomas.

Malignant melanomas appear as small-to-large brown-black or multicolored patches or nodules with irregular outlines that may crust on the surface or bleed. Very often, they arise in preexisting moles. If you notice any of these symptoms, you should visit a clinic or see a doctor immediately. Early detection could save your life. For this reason, the Skin Cancer Foundation has instituted skin cancer detection clinics in communities throughout the country, offering free skin checkups.

There is also an undeclared epidemic of other types of skin cancer, such as squamous and basal cell carcinoma. The American Cancer Society estimates that 700,000 Americans develop these more common types of skin cancer each year. While 99 percent of these cases are successfully treated, this is still a frightening statistic—and the number seems to be growing rapidly. The people most susceptible to these types of skin cancer are those who spend time directly exposed to sunlight. The cancerous nodules that occur most often on the face, hands, ears, neck, or other exposed areas of the body may crust, ulcerate, and sometimes bleed. Treatment by electrosurgery, excisional surgery, chemosurgery, cryosurgery, radiation, or chemotherapy usually cures these types of cancer, although reconstructive or corrective surgery may be required to restore the appearance of the skin's surface.

The rapid rise in incidence of skin cancers is blamed, by some, on damage to the atmospheric ozone layer, which serves as a natural protection against the sun's ultraviolet rays. For each 1 percent decrease in the ozone layer, it is estimated that certain types of skin cancers will increase 2 to

10 percent. The American Cancer Society estimates a decrease in the ozone layer of between 5 and 9 percent by the late twenty-first century.

Partial destruction of this vitally protective layer has been blamed on the use of fluorocarbons. In the 1970s, laws were passed banning their use in propellants and aerosol sprays, but by that time significant reduction of the layer had already taken place. Recent studies have not been able to determine whether the ban has had a meaningful impact. However, we do know that the hole in the ozone layer over the South Pole has increased in size, making daily incidental sun exposure in Australia and New Zealand potentially deadly. Australia has the highest incidence of skin cancer in the world, with two out of three Australians developing the disease. People in those countries have begun to take what just a few years ago would have been considered extreme precautions, such as staying indoors during prime sun hours (11:00 A.M. to 3:00 P.M.) and wearing various forms of high-tech sun protective clothing. School children are not allowed to play outside during school hours, and schools dispense sunscreen for their use. An extensive media campaign aimed at children warns: "Slip on a shirt, slop on a sunscreen, and slap on a hat!"

Another explanation for the increase in skin cancers is more frightening than ozone depletion: Two studies by researchers in the United States and Great Britain blame the rise in skin cancer on the use of PABA (para-aminobenzoic acid), the very substance used for many years to protect us from the sun. Experiments by Thomas Fitzpatrick, M.D., Ph.D., professor and chair, Department of Dermatology, Harvard University Medical School, showed that PABA caused mutagenic changes in the cells of mice. For this reason, for many years I have not recommended sunblocks containing PABA or its derivative, Padimate-O. Most companies have replaced this ingredient with less irritating and safer ones. However, any chemical designed to absorb ultraviolet light is potentially irritating to the skin, and any chemical consistently applied to the skin and then exposed to UV light may be potentially carcinogenic when used over an entire lifetime.

Sunblocks for Broad-Spectrum Protection

There are now a bewildering array of sunblock products on the market with sun protection factors (SPFs) ranging from 2 to 50. The SPF refers to how much longer a person wearing sunblock can stay in the sun before getting sunburned. If you have very fair skin and begin to burn in 15 minutes, using an SPF 4 sunblock would mean you could stay in the sun for an hour before burning. What most people don't realize is that reapplication of a sunscreen does not prolong the amount of time you can safely stay in the sun; an SPF 10 applied twice does not equal an SPF 20. The only reason to reapply a sunscreen is to replace any protection that may have been lost to perspiration or swimming.

Sunblocks are effective in protecting the skin, but what most people don't realize is that they only provide complete protection from the sun's UVB rays and protect only partially against harmful UVA rays. UVB rays, which are strongest in the summer, are composed of wavelengths from 290 to 320 nanometers and are responsible for physically burning the skin, thereby contributing to melanoma and other forms of skin cancer.

UVA rays are comprised of wavelengths between 320 and 400 nanometers and are relatively constant throughout the year. They are strongest in late afternoon. Once thought to be benign, they are now linked with skin aging, wrinkling, discoloration, and even skin cancer. These "aging rays" do not produce an immediate sunburn, but they do penetrate deep into the skin and damage the collagen and elastin fibers. Unlike UVB rays, UVA rays travel through clouds, fog, and haze and can even burn you on cloudy days. *They also penetrate glass*, which means that you are not safe while driving in your car or sitting by a sunny window. For these reasons, I always recommend choosing a sun protection product that guards against both UVB and UVA rays.

Currently, there is no approved rating system for UVA protection, which means that *the SPF on a product only reflects the protection you get against UVB rays.* In other words, three different sunblock products, each with an SPF 15, may each provide different UVA protection. Until a rating system for UVA rays is approved by the Food and Drug Administration, you simply cannot decipher a product's UVA protection ability. The only truly accurate way to know is to contact the manufacturer to find out the percentage of UVA blocker the product contains and how much of the UVA spectrum it blocks. See Chapter 14, "Product Information and Recommendations," for additional information about broad-spectrum sunblocks and about physical blocks that effectively protect against both UVA and UVB rays.

Many people use tanning salons, believing them to be a safe way to acquire a tan, but in fact, indoor tanning may be more dangerous than tanning under the sun. Tanning salons use only UVA rays, and often the dosage is several times stronger than the UVA in natural sunlight. In addition, a UVA tan does not protect against subsequent exposure to UVB rays. The UVA rays inhibit your body's natural repair process, which is needed to heal damage caused by UVB rays. This means that if you expose your skin to the sun following a salon tanning treatment, you will not have the benefit of your body's natural protective mechanism.

Needed: New Attitudes toward Sunning

Remember when we talked about having a "healthy tan"? It's difficult for many of us to accept that the sunshine we enjoy so much is skin enemy number one. Most of us love the feel of the sun on our bodies and think of a suntan as being both attractive and healthy. On vacation, we seek out the sun as an antidote to the stress of our daily lives, and the tan we return with is the badge we wear to indicate we had a relaxed, good time.

And let's not forget that the sun is good for us in several ways: It causes the body to produce vitamin D, necessary for strong bones; it inhibits the production of melatonin, the hormone responsible for decreasing the sex drive; it kills bacterial and fungal infections; and it is a mood elevator. Needless to say, without the sun we would not exist.

I am not suggesting that you avoid the sun completely, but rather that you protect yourself properly from its damaging effects *while you enjoy it.* Simple precautions can make a big difference—like wearing a broad-spectrum SPF 15 sunblock daily on the face, neck, and hands and applying it to the rest of your body when that is exposed. Wear a hat and sunglasses, and avoid prolonged, direct exposure to the sun between the hours of 10:00 A.M. and 3:00 P.M. A hat with a wide brim reduces your exposure by up to 70 percent, while avoiding midday sun saves you by 60 percent. The average cotton T-shirt has the equivalent of an SPF 10 to 15, while specially designed sun protective clothing will protect up to 99 percent. There's no need to make a big deal out of avoiding the sun; it just takes a little forethought. If you think of shunning sunning as a way to stay young and healthy, it seems to make the process very easy. In my anti-aging program in Chapter 13, I provide complete information for sensible daily sun care.

What to Do about Photoaged Skin

Don't despair if you have been a sun-worshipper all your life and are already seeing signs of damage. Take heart: *Cumulative sun damage is not irreversible.* One of the most encouraging developments of the past decade has been the fact that sun-damaged skin can be repaired and rejuvenated. Dr. Albert Kligman, M.D., Ph.D., the developer of Retin-A and the author of *Aging and the Skin,* states, "If you stay in the shade or use a sunblock, you will see a reversal of many of the changes in your skin. The connective tissue underneath will definitely improve. The fibroblasts have a chance to make new collagen. Precancerous lesions may disappear. After about two or three years of not being in the sun, you'll have what looks like a light peel, where a few of the upper layers of the skin have been removed, leaving the skin smooth-looking." The latest studies in Australia support this belief. In fact, one study successfully proved that protecting the skin from UV light by daily use of a sunscreen (SPF 16 or higher) allowed reversal of precancerous lesions, as well as prevention of new lesions.

Retin-A and Renova are touted as treatments for reversing sun damage, but experiments conducted at several universities to determine the effectiveness of these products came up with some surprising results. Patients in the placebo group—who received only sunblock, moisturizer, and instructions to stay out of the sun—showed subtle but perceptible improvement in the condition of their skin. The researchers concluded that using sunblock alone reduced the appearance of fine wrinkles, roughness, blotchiness, and uneven pigmentation. The sunblock itself was not responsible for the change, but by protecting the skin from further damage by ultraviolet light, the skin was allowed to heal itself.

The "before" and "after" pictures of me in this book's introduction demonstrate the reversal that is possible. As you will recall, at the time the "before" picture was taken in 1982, I had been a sun-worshipper for all of my 37 years. By 1994, not only had I been using my rejuvenating products for some time, but I had also eschewed sunning for 12 years. Had I continued to tan, I would look older than my age rather than younger.

Skin Enemy Number Two:
Internal and External Pollution

Remember those roving free radicals I talked about in Chapter 1—the real culprits in the aging process? Not only are free radicals increased by sun damage, they are also the result of such factors as drug use, cigarette smoke, alcohol abuse, stress, inadequate diet, various forms of environmental toxins, and certain medications like antibiotics. All of these factors affect cell oxidation in the body, and free-radical damage to healthy cells is increased when there are not enough antioxidants to neutralize them.

I realize that there are some types of pollution you just can't avoid if you live in a city, drive on the freeway, or work in a closed, central air system building. In these places, air pollution is going to take its toll as long as you have to keep breathing. But there are some forms of internal and external pollution that can and should be avoided if you want your skin to stay young.

Cigarette smoking, which is known to be dangerous to health, is one of the worst enemies of the skin. Smoking is second only to sunlight as an aging factor. It impairs the circulation of blood to the skin, depriving it of nutrients and oxygen and causing severe dehydration. It also depletes the body of vitamins A, E, C, and B complex, and the minerals calcium, potassium, and zinc. One cigarette uses up 25 milligrams of vitamin C. The place where these deficiencies show most obviously is the face. Cigarette smokers develop severe premature wrinkling, crepeyness, and bags and dark circles under the eyes. A recent study shows that the skin of smokers ages almost twice as fast as that of nonsmokers, after age 30. And, as if this nutrient deprivation isn't enough, the puckering of the lips and squinting of the eyes involved in the act of smoking create even more facial lines.

The effects of *alcohol abuse* are very similar to those of cigarette smoking. They share the same nutrient-robbing and dehydrating properties, and both damage the blood and internal organs, especially the liver. When the liver is not functioning properly, it shows on the skin in the form of a sallow, dead appearance. A more noticeable effect of heavy alcohol consumption is the reddening of the skin on the face, caused by the dilation of blood vessels. This is commonly referred to as the "blush effect." Eventually the pores on the nose and cheeks also become enlarged.

You may not be a smoker or drinker, but you will still have vitamin-deficient skin if you have an *inadequate diet*, or if you indulge in crash dieting. Trying every new fad diet that hits the market can do just as much harm to the skin as it can to the metabolism. Some of these diets produce nutrient deprivation, which can cause serious harm as well as death. The "Beverly Hills Diet," which consisted solely of fruits, lacked protein as well as fats. During the height of its popularity, I treated many people for excessively dry skin and scalp, and several who had begun to lose their hair. Protein deprivation is a serious health problem that can permanently affect a person's metabolism. Prolonged fasting or long juice fasts can have a similar effect. The skin may become dehydrated, flaky, or sallow. And consider the results of continual stretching and shrinking. Skin stretches to accommodate weight gain, then shrinks during weight loss. After a few years of this pattern, the skin loses its elasticity and begins to sag. This is true for skin all over the body, not just on the face!

Avoiding Environmental Toxins

There is a great deal of discussion and debate going on about the impact of environmental pollution on skin aging. While we have not yet seen much scientific evidence that pollution damages skin, a growing number of dermatologists believe there is a link—based on their own experiences with patients. More and more people are seeing their doctors for problems such as skin dryness, inflammation, irritation, and increased sensitivity. What accounts for this new rash of skin problems?

We do know that free-radical production is triggered by environmental toxins and that smog, automobile exhaust, dirt, and smoke are being absorbed daily by the skin. Pollutants trapped in air-conditioning systems of buildings can also end up on and in the skin. Some researchers suspect that electromagnetic radiation from the screens of computer terminals is linked to a problem called "rosacea," a skin condition that causes redness, sensitivity, and sometimes breakouts on the face.

All this might sound like a good excuse to avoid going to work, but few of us can afford that option. The importance of good skin care takes on a new dimension in this age of ozone depletion, environmental pollution, and increasing on-the-job hazards. The name of the game becomes "protection"—from the inside as well as the outside of the body.

Menopause and the Skin

Another important factor in skin aging for women is the onset of menopause, that time in a woman's life when her body stops manufacturing estrogen and when ovulation and menstruation cease. Menopause is a rite of passage now affecting millions of women in the baby boom generation, and for the first time in history, this transition is being talked about, written about, and studied extensively. While much information about menopause remains to be discovered, the subject is at least out in the open, and we can benefit from its new acceptance and widespread discussion. We can also appreciate that "The Change" is not just a physical or biological event, but one that has profound personal, emotional, and social ramifications as well.

The impact of menopause of the lives of women varies greatly: Some women find the transition "no big deal," whereas others find themselves suffering months, perhaps years, of physical and emotional discomfort. Symptoms can appear at any time in what is technically called "the perio-menopausal process": *premenopause,* when periods become irregular and lighter or heavier; *menopause,* when the periods stop; and *postmenopause.* The process can begin in the early forties or in the early fifties, but by age 55, 95 percent of women will be postmenopausal.

We are all becoming aware of the potential physical problems of menopause—conditions such as hot flashes, headaches, heart palpitations, fatigue, insomnia, weight gain, dry skin, hair loss, and vaginal dryness that can mean painful intercourse. Emotionally, there can be increased anxiety, irritability, "fuzzy-mindedness," changes in sexual drive, and mild to deep depression, which can compound the stress in women's lives. On top of all this, there can be women's increasing concern about their physical appearance and general attractiveness and the fear of "looking old."

This book cannot address all the potential physical and emotional problems of menopause, but it's important to consider what is happening during this change in order to understand how to prevent and deal with menopausal-related skin changes The hormonal changes that take place during menopause do affect the skin—though compared to other problems, dry skin and occasional acne can seem like the least of your worries!

Still, for many women, the wrinkles that begin to seem more apparent as they enter menopause are the most visible, tangible signs of aging. There are also other skin changes that are hormonally related—increased dryness, loss of skin elasticity, and, for many women, the appearance or reappearance of acne. Usually activated by hormone change, acne can show up during puberty, pregnancy, and menopause. I will discuss the treatment of acne in Chapter 10, "A Holistic Approach to Problem Skin."

Hormones: To Replace or Not to Replace . . .

Many women are attracted to hormone replacement therapy in hopes of achieving younger-looking skin. Hormone replacement therapy, or HRT, refers to replacing the estrogen and progesterone depleted by menopause. Whether to take hormones or not is one of the most confusing questions facing menopausal women. We have heard about the benefits of taking estrogen—protection against heart disease and osteoporosis, as well as the relief of hot flashes and other symptoms. But we have also heard about the link between estrogen and breast cancer or uterine cancer. Some doctors are enthusiastic about hormone replacement therapy and recommend it to their menopausal patients, whereas others are skeptical and prescribe it only under dire circumstances.

In the 1950s and 1960s, only estrogen was prescribed for menopausal women, and by the mid-1970s, reports were indicating that women on long-term estrogen replacement were showing increased evidence of endometrial cancer (cancer of the lining of the uterus). HRT fell out of favor until it was confirmed that adding progesterone to the formula would effectively protect against cancer. Now, doctors are once again prescribing HRT, and while there is still discussion of the impact of estrogen on breast cancer, the most recent studies indicate that risk is diminished when estrogen and progesterone are taken together.

Does HRT really affect skin aging? Lonnie Barbach, author of *The Pause: Positive Approaches to Menopause*, states, "While supplemental estrogen does not seem to be the fountain of youth for the skin that it was purported to be when it first came on the market, it does tend to make the skin a little plumper and reduce excess dryness both by increasing skin collagen and by holding moisture in the skin." There is anecdotal evidence that taking hormones has a positive effect on the skin, but I know of only one study that seems to prove it. An experiment conducted at Laval University in Quebec, Canada, did show that postmenopausal women who were given estrogen showed increased thickness of the skin as compared to similar women not taking estrogen.

Deciding whether or not to take hormones and for how long is a very individual decision that should not be made only on the basis of skin appearance. It is a decision to be made in consultation with your doctor, hopefully a physician who is knowledgeable about menopause and HRT and who also has the patience and care to deal with you on an individual basis. There are different kinds of hormones, both synthetically and naturally derived, and a number of ways to take them—orally, vaginally, rubbing them into the skin, or via a skin patch. There are also various combinations of hormones to be taken according to different regimens. You may need to experiment with various forms of HRT before you discover what—if anything—works for you.

Menopausal Treatment Alternatives

One of the newest developments in menopausal treatment is the use of natural forms of estrogen and progesterone. They are derived from soybeans and wild Mexican yams and delivered transdermally by massaging a cream into the skin. The creams may also be used intravaginally. There are few reported side effects from either. Many health practitioners are finding that the progesterone cream alone helps relieve menopausal symptoms and is an effective alternative to hormone replacement therapy.

Menopausal women are also finding that ancient Chinese herbal remedies like dong quai and ginseng, as well as other plants, relieve hot flashes and vaginal dryness. There are quite a few other alternatives to hormonal supplements available through acupuncturists, homeopaths, and herbalists who are knowledgeable about menopause. These treatments may be useful for those of you who don't want to take hormones or who have reacted badly to taking them. See the Recommended Reading section for a list of books on natural approaches to menopause. Also, keep in mind that diet, exercise, and relaxation have a great deal to do with how you experience menopause. Recommendations for diet modification and supplementation, fitness, and anti-stress are discussed in Chapters 4, 5, 6, and 9.

Aging: What Is Inevitable? What Can Be Prevented?

If we examine the factors that contribute to aging skin—exposure to sunlight, primarily, as well as substances we consume, products we use, environmental toxins, and mental attitude—it is evident that *the aging of our skin is something that is very much under our control.*

The only aging factor we can't do anything about is *genetics.* As noted, your ethnic or racial background figures prominently in how your skin responds to photoaging. If you are blond and fair-skinned, you will have to take much greater care in the sun than if you are African-American or Asian. Genetic aging also occurs as a result of facial expressions. You may very well have the same frown, grimace, or grin as one of your parents or grandparents and therefore create the same patterns of facial lines. You may also have some of the same bad habits as your parents or grandparents, such as smoking cigarettes, drinking too much alcohol, or eating an unhealthy diet. Your skin also tends to accumulate fat in the same way as that of your forebears: If your mother (or grandmother) has jowls or a double chin, your face may follow suit.

But genetics play a far less significant role in skin aging than most of us think. Sorry, we can't blame mom or dad for those wrinkles; more likely, it was all those years of cultivating an unhealthy tan. The fact that saving your skin is up to you should be very good news indeed! The rest of this book will tell you all you need to know to take responsibility for your skin and improve its condition, as well as improve your general health. For the ultimate anti-aging program is not just looking young on the outside, but staying fit and healthy from the inside out.

4

Beauty from the Inside Out: The Anti-Aging Way of Eating

Look at it this way: What you put *in* your face is just as important as what you put *on* your face. The old adage "You are what you eat" is literally true when it comes to your skin.

The way your skin looks reveals a great deal about your general body health. In fact, many doctors and alternative health practitioners can diagnose health problems simply by looking at a person's skin. You may know this from your own experience. Picture someone you know who is over 40 and unhealthy. Maybe this person is a heavy smoker or drinker and doesn't exercise or eat properly. Now visualize that person's skin. It's probably not a pretty picture. Even when a healthy friend is under stress, we can often see it in his or her skin—sallowness, breakouts, undereye puffiness, or dark circles.

Since the skin renews itself every four weeks, it is very responsive to what is going on inside the body. Very simply, the quality of the skin reflects the quality of the raw materials used to make cells. Makeup can cover some signs of an unhealthy lifestyle, but ultimately the ravages of poor diet, no exercise, stress, and lack of sleep will become apparent no matter how good the makeup job.

Since healthy, vibrant skin is a reflection of a healthy, vibrant body, the way to look younger throughout life is to work *from the inside out*. The most important aspect of a program of good health is what you put into your body on a daily basis. This means the food you eat as well as vitamins and supplements that build up your immune system and combat aging. It may also involve periodic detoxification of the body so that you make the most of eating a healthy diet.

If you don't already know that you should be eating a lowfat, low-cholesterol, high-fiber diet, you probably haven't been living on Planet Earth the past several years. The glut of information, opinion, and warnings about the food we eat is often completely overwhelming. Perhaps that's why so many people choose to ignore it and continue to consume Big Macs, fries, and shakes. Even those of us who want to do what's right for our bodies foodwise can become so confused by conflicting advice that we may subconsciously rebel—feel like grabbing a hamburger and forgetting about it.

Avoiding the Fad-Diet Trap

Eating a healthy diet is not "dieting." If you switch from a diet high in fat, starch, and sugar to a healthful diet, you will most likely lose weight. But thinness should not be the goal of your way of eating, it should be the by-product.

As we know, Americans are obsessed with dieting, making diet books the consistent best-sellers in this country. Unfortunately, a thin body is primarily what people want from these diets—not good health. Even health-oriented diet books, such as *Fit for Life* and the *Pritikin Diet*, offer thinness as an added benefit to good health. Fortunately, the American medical community agrees that a thin person stands a greater chance of being healthy than does a fat person.

Some diet fads may have helped people lose weight, but have had unhealthy side effects. Several years ago, a high-protein diet was considered good for supplying energy and burning excess fat. Then it was discovered that most Americans consume more protein than they need. If the protein consumed came from an animal source, it meant high cholesterol, which is bad for the blood and heart. Then liquid protein diets, which avoided the pitfalls of animal protein, became the vogue, but fell into disfavor when they were blamed for several deaths (resulting from the failure to supply other necessary nutrients, specifically selenium and potassium). Fruit-based diets have always been popular with people interested in quick weight loss and inner cleansing of the body; but staying on a fruit-only diet for too long can cause protein deprivation, which leads to hair loss, headaches, physical and mental weakness, and more serious maladies, including death. Going off the fruit or liquid protein diets and resuming a diet that includes a variety of foods usually causes the weight to return.

Fortunately, dieters now have sensible, healthy options for losing weight—particularly the high-carbohydrate diet that became popular a few years ago. It was welcomed with particular enthusiasm by those who for years had been denying themselves foods such as pasta and potatoes.

The sad but true news about dieting, however, is that it rarely works. About 90 to 95 percent of the people who go on diets regain the weight they had lost within a few months. *The only way to keep weight off is to permanently change your way of eating.* Rather than going on a diet again and again, you need to find a way of eating that is varied, enjoyable, and that suits your personal lifestyle. Good eating habits can become effortless and interesting with time, rather than tedious and boring like most diets. And the more you learn about incorporating beneficial, healthful foods into your everyday life, the more choices are available, and the more enjoyable and rewarding healthful eating becomes.

A healthy body and young-looking skin depend on a balanced diet of nutritious, unprocessed foods including fruits and vegetables, high fiber from whole grains, adequate protein, and lots of water. These foods keep the body functioning at its peak and fight the breakdowns that are associated with age and illness. When you eat a proper diet, the organs do their jobs, the blood carries necessary nutrients and oxygen to cells and organs, and toxins are released rather than stored.

10 Basic Rules for Anti-Aging Eating

Instead of recommending a specific diet for you to follow to stay healthy and young looking, my aim is to provide you with the basic guidelines you need to begin discovering your own healthful, satisfying, and creative way to eat. Following these 10 Basic Rules of Anti-Aging Eating will enable you to have the body you want, to live longer, and to enjoy excellent health that will show up on your skin.

1. Eat Plenty of Fiber.

Fiber is one of the most important cleansers of the body because it is not absorbed during digestion. It passes through your digestive tract, taking with it undigested waste that can otherwise impede digestion and poison your body. The more effectively your body processes what you eat, the fewer problems you will have. The faster food moves through your intestines, the less time there is for fat to be absorbed by your body. When dietary fiber is lacking, body waste sits in the colon where bioacids and bacteria concentrate. The water in the stool is reabsorbed back into the body along with toxins, and the stool becomes hard and dry. This is why lack of fiber is linked to hemorrhoids, constipation, and colon cancer.

Research has also proven that a high-fiber diet is one of the best preventatives against heart disease, arteriosclerosis, colon cancer, breast cancer, and diabetes. Fiber also slows the absorption of sugar to help regulate blood insulin levels.

You can barely listen to a TV food commercial these days without hearing something about fiber. You would think that Americans are eating it by the ton, but we are barely beginning to return to the fiber levels of 80 to 100 years ago. The average American consumes about 15 grams of fiber a day. The National Cancer Institute recommends 25 to 30 grams a day.

There are two main types of fiber: pectin and cellulose. Pectin is found primarily in fruits and vegetables and helps to break up cholesterol in the blood. Cellulose, found predominantly in the bran of whole grains such as oat and wheat, aids the passage of foods through the intestines. Some good sources of fiber are raw bran, oats, whole-wheat cereals and breads, wheat berries, dry beans and peas, raw apples, raw carrots, almonds, spinach, broccoli, cabbage, and celery.

If your diet has been lacking in fiber and you want to get more immediately, you can take fiber supplements such as Fibercon and Crystal Star Chol-Lo Fiber Tone. These are excellent fiber sources, but should not be permanently substituted for the real thing—fiber in foods. Think about your diet and see where you can add more fibrous foods. Red meats, chicken, and fish contain no fiber at all; dietary fiber is found only in the leaves, stems, flowers, tubers, roots, and seeds of plant foods. To preserve the fiber and nutrients in fruits and vegetables, leave the skin on when possible and cook lightly by steaming or sautéing. Beans are a very good source of fiber and should be increasingly incorporated into your diet. And keep in mind that white flour and white rice contain no fiber—it was removed from the grain during processing.

2. Eat a Lowfat Diet.

While we do need some fat in our diet, most of us consume far too much in proportion to other types of foods. Eating too much fat is not only what makes us fat, it is also a major cause of heart disease, which kills more Americans than all other diseases combined. Hardened fat clogs veins, making the passage of blood difficult and eventually impossible. The heart must work harder and harder to pump blood and then it gives up in a heart attack.

Government guidelines for fat consumption have improved over the past few years, but, from my perspective, they are still too high. Nutritionists believe that instead of the 30 percent of calories from fat that is currently recommended, you should consume about 15 to 20 percent, which for the average woman is between 25 and 40 grams per day.

To reduce the amount of fat in your diet, start at the top of the food chain. Animal fat is the highest source of saturated fats and cholesterol—particularly that found in red meat. If you do eat red meat occasionally, choose lean cuts over fatty ones and trim excess fat before cooking. Alternatives to red meat, of course, are chicken (without the fatty skin) and fish. Eating fish in place of meat is an excellent idea for more reasons than cutting down on fat. Fish supplies oils called omega 3 and omega 6 that help break up (reduce) cholesterol. It is also high in vitamin A, a potent antioxidant and nutrient.

Another source of fat is dairy products—milk, butter, and cheese. You do not need to eliminate them entirely from your diet, because they are a good source of many nutrients, but you should consume them in their lowest fat form. If you like milk, drink nonfat or skim milk instead of whole, and replace cream with lowfat milk. Choose nonfat yogurt, cottage cheese, sour cream, and cream cheese instead of regular. Cut down on the amount of cheese in your diet, and use butter very sparingly. Margarine is really not much of an improvement over butter, since it too can affect serum cholesterol. Eggs also are a source of cholesterol, and it is now suggested that you eat only a few eggs a week, or opt for cholesterol-free egg products (made from egg whites). Personally, I have found it easy to switch to using only egg whites at all times. They make great omelettes and scrambles and work just as well in most recipes as whole eggs.

We all need a small amount of oil in our diet to keep moisture in the skin. Beware, however, of the amount and type of oil you consume. Saturated oils (such as palm and coconut) and hydrogenated oil (like vegetable shortening) clog veins and arteries; like animal fat, these oils are the worst for your body. They are particularly bad for your skin, making cell membranes less porous so that nutrients can't get in and wastes can't get out. Monosaturated oils like olive and canola are the best alternatives; there is evidence that they may even help protect the heart. They are also available in cooking sprays, which make it easy to cut down on the amount you use without sacrificing flavor.

3. Build Your Diet Around Complex Carbohydrates.

If you want to increase your fiber and lower your fat, what do you eat? The answer is complex carbohydrates. To have good energy available to your body, you must eat carbohydrates, and complex carbohydrates are the body's main fuel source. They burn slowly and do not contain fat. Because they have a lot of fiber, they stay in the body longer. As a result, you feel fuller longer, your blood sugar stays more even, and your energy level and mood are more stable.

The major portion of your diet should consist of complex carbohydrates, which include fruits, vegetables, rice, pasta, grains, breads, beans, nuts, and seeds. You may want to experiment with some of the less common grains, such as buckwheat groats (kasha), couscous, and millet. They are delicious and can be used in a wide variety of dishes, from "veggie burgers" to cereals and pilaf. Whole grains supply both zinc, a nutrient that is critical to skin health, and essential fatty acids, which keep the skin moist, smooth, and soft and prevent pores from clogging. Beans abound in dozens of varieties and can be used in hundreds of ways, including soups, stews, casseroles, loaves, spreads, side dishes, and dips. If you have a hard time digesting beans, try

Beano, a commercially sold product that can be added to bean dishes or to any gas-producing food. Or, you can try this tip from master chef Dorah Carllyn of New York City: Soak a strip of kombu seaweed in water until soft, then add to your pot of beans while they cook.

We distinguish between complex carbohydrates and simple carbohydrates, which are processed foods such as white flour, white rice, and refined sugar. In the processing, fiber, vitamins, and minerals are removed, leaving a quick-burning energy source without many nutrients. Even "enriched" flours and cereals can't compare to the "whole" version—about 20 nutrients are taken out and only a few are added back in.

4. Eat Fresh, Locally Grown, Organic Foods.

The fresher the food, the better it is for your body. Food that is processed or stored for long periods of time loses nutrients and may also contain chemicals added to preserve a "fresh" appearance. In fact, most fruits and vegetables are picked long before they are ripe, then stored for varying lengths of time before delivery to stores. Apples may be stored for as long as a year!

One principle to follow in creating a healthy diet is to eat foods that are in season and are organically grown near where you live. This is a tall order and may be some-what difficult, but now that health food stores are fairly ubiquitous you can probably easily find organic produce as well as grains, breads, and cereals. Local farmers markets and roadside produce stands are good sources for produce that is fresh and ripe, and often for organically raised produce.

While it may seem wonderful to have strawberries in December and peaches in February, think about where these fruits come from. In many other countries, pesticide laws are not as strict as ours. The use of DDT is banned in the United States, but it is still sold to other countries and may come back to us from Latin America, for example, in grapes, bananas, and coffee.

Although organic produce is usually more expensive than commercially raised produce, it tastes so much better that many think it's worth the extra cost. You might also consider the costs of nonorganic eating: Pesticides, mercury, and other toxins cause oxidation in cells, remain in the body, and can cause cancer. Keep in mind also that as demand for organic food grows, the prices will come down!

If you can't get organic fruits and vegetables, be sure to wash the commercial variety before eating. To thoroughly remove toxins from the skins of vegetables and fruits, soak them for 10 minutes in a large bowl of water to which you have added a few drops of liquid bleach.

5. Keep Sugar and Salt to a Minimum.

In the average American's diet, salt is consumed in a quantity measured at approximately 10 to 25 times more than necessary. For basic good health, the body requires about 250 milligrams of salt a day, as opposed to the 2500 to 8000 milligrams consumed by most Americans.

Excess salt is detrimental to the body because it contributes to high blood pressure, which in turn puts a terrible strain on the body and can eventually cause it to break down permanently. Salt is also responsible for water retention, which not only causes bloating, swelling of joints, and puffy eyes but accentuates cellulite.

The most obvious way to cut down on the amount of salt in your diet is to stop adding it to your food. You'll be surprised at how sensitive you become to the taste of salt after just a few weeks without it. Also, take a good look at the processed foods you normally eat. Read the labels for sodium content and you'll be amazed at the amount of salt these products contain. The biggest offenders are cereals, crackers, soups, and snack foods. It's easy to replace these salt-laden products with their salt-free counterparts.

Sugar is also greatly overused in our society. The average American consumes over 100 pounds a year—this averages out to 5 ounces per person per day! It's not hard to see how this happens when you realize that one cola drink contains 12 teaspoons of sugar or corn syrup, which, by the way, is just as bad as refined sugar.

We all know that sugar is a factor in tooth decay, but we are just beginning to discover its role in various other diseases. Recent studies conducted at the United States Drug Administration's Human Nutrition Center have shown that sugar raises the serum cholesterol, triglyceride, and insulin levels in adults. Men who have difficulty metabolizing carbohydrates are especially prone to these problems. Sugar may also play a role in other health problems because, when consumed in large quantities, it replaces other nutrients needed for good health.

There are a number of other sweeteners that will allow you to cut down on the amount of refined sugar in your diet. You can use honey, maple syrup, molasses, rice syrup, or sucanat (made from raw sugar cane juice). For desserts, substitute fresh fruit, raisins, dried dates, figs, or apricots. If these sound too boring, natural food stores usually stock a wide variety of puddings, cakes, and cookies made with alternative natural sweeteners and healthy ingredients. One of my favorites is Chocolate Dream Pudding, which is both sugar and fat free. You can even buy sugar-free nut fudge that is heavenly! Natural, sugarless chewing gum or hard candies may also satisfy a sweet craving.

If you are a heavy sugar user, giving up this addictive substance may not be so easy. You may want to read *Sugar Blues* by William Dufty for inspiration and insight into sugar addiction.

6. Eat More Nonanimal Protein Than Animal Protein.

Protein is crucial to body health, both as a source of energy and because proteins form our muscles, hormones, enzymes, and antibodies.

One of the major problems with the American diet is that when we think of protein, we think of red meats, chicken, fish, or dairy products. Thus, the average American diet relies too heavily on animal protein, which is not only high in saturated fat and cholesterol, but may also contain other toxic substances—growth hormones, antibiotics, and pesticides contained in commercial feeds. Unfortunately, when we cut down on our meat consumption, we tend to eat more cheese, which is also high in saturated fat.

We need to focus our protein consumption on more nonanimal sources such as complex carbohydrates. Did you know that a cup of broccoli contains 2.6 grams of protein? Beans and legumes are also rich in protein, as are tofu products, nuts, and seeds. Bear in mind that most of us eat more protein than we really need. The average woman needs 1 gram of protein for every kilogram of body weight—about 40 to 60 grams per day.

Combining foods the right way can boost the protein value of nonanimal foods such as beans and rice. This is an interesting as well as tasty approach to getting the usable protein you need. For a fascinating explanation of food-combining as well as great recipes, see the latest edition of the classic book *Diet for a Small Planet*.

7. Give Up Caffeine.

If you want your skin to look its best, you're going to have to give up caffeine. Caffeine causes severe dehydration of the skin because it depletes vitamins and oxygen. It robs the body of the exact nutrients needed to create collagen and new skin cells as well as those needed to fight free-radical damage (vitamins A, C, E, and zinc). Tea, which has approximately half as much caffeine as coffee, contains tannin, which impedes the absorption of iron. When these vital nutrients are low, energy levels drop and stress levels rise. The vascular constriction caused by caffeine causes circulation to slow down. This restricts the flow of blood to facial muscles, depriving them of the oxygen and nutrients they need to stay healthy and strong.

Too much caffeine stresses the hormonal system and blood sugar metabolism. The body releases adrenaline, which raises the blood sugar, then the pancreas sends in glucose to bring it down. As this happens over and over again, the adrenal glands get tired and begin to "need" the caffeine to function. This is why caffeine is so addicting. Need I say more? If you are using caffeine as an energy source, to get you going and keep you going when you're tired, consider just paying attention to your body and giving it what it *really* wants—perhaps more sleep, relaxation, or exercise.

You can train yourself to enjoy decaffeinated coffee and tea as well as the many wonderful herbal teas now available. If you do drink a cup of caffeinated coffee, be sure to follow it with two glasses of water to help replenish the skin.

If you want to go "cold turkey" to wean yourself from caffeine, it will take you about three weeks. The heavier the addiction, the more severe the withdrawal. You will most probably have headaches for several days. It's fine to take ibuprofen, aspirin, or whatever you would normally take for headache pain. You can also count on being tired, and possibly even needing to nap occasionally. Some people report feeling slightly depressed and/or irritable. When I went through this, I wanted to strangle anyone who crossed my line of sight! But stick it out and soon you'll be free of the caffeine habit for good. When several months have gone by (and your skin looks so much better), drink a cup of coffee and see what happens. I'll bet it will be your last cup ever!

When you quit using caffeine, it's advisable to take the following supplements for 8 to 12 weeks:

◆ Take large doses of vitamin C (1 gram every two to three hours, because the body doesn't store it), which helps to flush caffeine from the body and increase the percentage of calcium that is absorbed. Try a buffered one, which is less likely to upset your stomach.

◆ Double up on B complex by taking 100 milligrams twice daily.

◆ A calcium–magnesium supplement will help to calm your nerves. A total of 2500 milligrams, taken between meals and at bedtime, is recommended.

◆ A daily dosage of 30 milligrams of zinc (15 milligrams with one meal, 15 milligrams with another) will help replace what your body has lost.

By the way, caffeine is also a prime irritant for women with benign fibrocystic breast disease. When caffeine is eliminated, the painful nodules and symptoms usually disappear.

8. Avoid Artificial Food Enhancers.

Artificial food enhancers include artificial sweeteners, flavors, and colors; preservatives; and the "taste enhancers," monosodium glutamate (MSG) and hydrolyzed vegetable protein. The average American consumes 7 to 12 pounds of preservatives and food additives a year! Since the body is unable to process many of these substances, they accumulate in fat, joints, and organs. Artificial flavors and preservatives can cause skin breakouts, and artificial sweeteners can cause joint pain and arthritic-like symptoms. Some have even been shown to be carcinogenic in large doses. Sulfites, commonly used in wine and to keep salad-bar ingredients fresh, can trigger asthma and respiratory problems. MSG and hydrolyzed vegetable protein (which has the same chemical composition as MSG) can have a wide range of effects on the body, even in very small amounts. Those who are sensitive report joint and neck pain, migraine headaches, nervous tension, or even serious emotional symptoms such as anger, depression, and hysteria. Since most symptoms don't occur until 24 to 48 hours after consumption, many people don't make the connection between the cause and the effects.

Keep in mind that while there are over 6000 substances on the government's GRAS (generally accepted as safe) list, they have all been tested separately. No one knows what the effects of combining several food additives might be. The best way to avoid these substances is to eat fresh, unprocessed foods. If you are sensitive to MSG, make sure to read all processed-food labels carefully, because it is used in everything from soups to salad dressings to frozen spinach soufflé. Also inquire in restaurants about whether they use it or not; most Chinese and Japanese restaurants add it to their dishes.

9. Drink Six Glasses of Water Daily.

Keeping the body flushed with water not only helps eliminate wastes and toxins, it is also highly beneficial to the skin. Nothing will help your skin look younger than good hydration, which means sufficient water content; the best way to hydrate skin is from the inside out. Think of the difference between a ripe plum and a dried prune: The only difference is water. If your skin is dehydrated, it can look like a dried prune—dull, lifeless, and wrinkled.

If you drink at least six glassfuls of pure water every day, you will see a real improvement in your skin. The quality of the water is important, however. In general, tap water can contain chemicals, toxins, and even bacteria that you don't want in your body. Recent reports about the contamination of our cities' water supplies are very disturbing.

Thirty percent of cities tested showed serious contamination problems.

Make sure the water you drink is either purchased pure (bottled distilled or mineral water, carbonated or non-carbonated, as you wish) or is run through a home water purifier. If you choose mineral water, pick a brand with a low sodium content, or you could experience bloating (water retention). Contrary to what you might think, drinking a lot of water does not cause bloating. In fact, it has a diuretic effect on the body and helps remove toxins and waste very efficiently.

10. If You Drink Alcohol, Do So Only in Moderation.

Alcohol is a major cause of oxidation in cells; it also causes constriction of blood vessels, which carry nutrients and oxygen to cells. As well as directly damaging the liver, alcohol dehydrates the body and robs it of the vitamins, trace elements, and minerals necessary for it to function properly. Light to moderate alcohol consumption is considered acceptable by most doctors and nutritionists. In fact, many recommend a glass or two of wine daily as protection against heart disease. The speculation is that wine helps to build red blood cells as well as reduce bad cholesterol. Wine is also high in chromium, one of the elements that fights heart disease. But remember that most wines contain sulfites, which can trigger asthma and respiratory problems.

One or two ounces of hard liquor, such as scotch or vodka, is also considered acceptable, but for some people this is too much. Regardless of what the norm may be, getting to know what works best for *you* is the key. It is important to know that women are far more sensitive to the toxic effects of alcohol than men. Some researchers have found that as little as two drinks a week can upset a woman's hormonal balance. Anecdotal evidence seems to indicate that menopausal and postmenopausal women become more sensitive to the effects of alcohol.

Several new studies seem to show a link between alcohol consumption and breast cancer. It is now believed that women who consume even moderate amounts (as few as three drinks a week) may be somewhat more at risk than women who do not drink at all. Fourteen out of 17 studies conducted by National Cancer Research scientists, in collaboration with researchers at other institutes, support these findings. Results were published in the *New England Journal of Medicine* on May 7, 1987. Women at risk should be most concerned and may want to curtail their consumption of alcohol.

If you are going to drink alcohol, it's important to replace the nutrients that will be lost. On an evening in which you've had a drink or two, take the following vitamins with a spoonful of yogurt and a large glass of water before going to bed, and again the next morning with breakfast: vitamin E, 800 I.U.; vitamin C, 100 mg; B complex, 100 mg; calcium/magnesium, 1000 mg.

If you have a problem with alcohol, you will of course need to cut way back on drinking and begin a program of detoxification and vitamin supplements to counter the damaging effects of alcohol abuse. A doctor or nutritionist with a holistic approach can design a program to fit your needs.

These 10 rules are meant as general guidelines for a healthy diet. To create a program that is geared to your individual needs, you may need further research and perhaps consultation with a nutritionist. There are many resources for learning about what constitutes a healthy diet, and I hope you will consult them for more in-depth information. Again, the more you know, the more enjoyable and interesting the challenge of living a healthy life becomes.

Restoring the Body through Detoxification

If you are just beginning a program of physical health—abandoning the sedentary life, taking up exercise, and changing your diet—you may want to incorporate into that a program of detoxification of your body. Even if you feel your lifestyle is healthy and balanced, you can benefit from a periodic detoxification to ensure that you get the most benefit from healthy diet and exercise. If you are retaining water or toxins, you will never achieve optimal body tone by exercise alone. Water retention and toxic pollution must also be treated from the inside.

Toxins and toxic wastes that remain in the body are harmful in two ways: First, they start chemical reactions that ultimately produce free radicals; second, the body's defense mechanisms surround the toxins with fluids and fats in an attempt to render them harmless. These globules of "protected" toxins form the basis of the lumps and bumps we know as cellulite. To rid your body of toxins, you need to cleanse it at the level of the organs. This means cleansing the digestive tract and replacing bacteria in the intestines as well as cleansing and oxygenating the blood. In actuality, it's a lot simpler than it sounds.

Cleansing the Intestinal Tract

Maintaining a high fiber content in your diet is the best way to avoid constipation and ensure proper function of the intestinal tract. Regardless of how healthy your diet is, however, some substances stubbornly cling to the inner walls of the intestines. Taking a laxative or simply eating a bowl of bran will not dislodge this "sludge."

Several methods are used to clean the intestinal tract. The easiest is a "psyllium seed flush." Psyllium is a tiny seed that may be purchased in health food stores. It comes in either whole seed form or only the husks. When mixed with water, the seeds turn into a swollen, gelatinous glob, which travels through the intestines, taking with it any waste clinging to the intestinal walls. Mix three tablespoons of whole psyllium seeds with a few ounces of your favorite juice and drink it. Follow this with a large glass of water. Do this three times a day for two days. On the third day, drink the same amount twice, and on the fourth and fifth days, drink the same amount once. This is a very gentle yet effective flush that can be repeated every few months. For most people it does not cause cramping, bloating, diarrhea, or discomfort. On the third or fourth day you can expect one or two large bowel movements, which will carry out all the old intestinal sludge. This cleansing method may be done two to three times a year to help maintain the health and function of your intestines.

Replacing Intestinal Bacteria

Even moderate consumption of meat, alcohol, chemicals, sugar, and caffeine kills off the friendly intestinal bacteria necessary for digestion and assimilation of nutrients. These bacteria are called *Lactobacillus acidophilus, Lactobacillus bifidus, Lactobacillus bulgaricus*, and *Lactobacillus caucasicus*. Frequent indigestion or bloating after meals can be a sign of a lack of these bacteria. Constipation and blemishes also can go hand in hand with these symptoms as a result of the body's inability to digest food properly.

To begin replenishing the various types of lactobacilli in your intestinal tract, you can take a product that contains a living strain of these bacteria. This can be found in a powder, liquid, or capsule form at your local health food store. The refrigerated types are usually the most potent. In general, I recommend that you take lactobacillus for two or three weeks as follows: powder or liquid, three tablespoonsful before each meal and at bedtime; capsule, two before each meal and at bedtime.

Most people respond quickly and positively to this simple treatment and repeat it several times a year to ensure that intestinal balance is being maintained. As you become more familiar with your body, you'll know when you need lactobacillus. By the way, it also makes a much better instant antidote for simple indigestion than an antacid. Just take three tablespoonsful of the liquid when indigestion occurs. After following this treatment, if your digestion is still sluggish, you may need to further decrease the amounts of foods that are destructive to bacteria. If your digestion still does not improve, check with a doctor or nutritionist. You may lack hydrochloric acid in your stomach, or have some other condition that should be treated professionally.

Cleansing and Oxygenating the Blood

The cleaner and more oxygen-rich the blood, the more efficient and productive the cells and muscles. In principle, the way the human body works is not that different from the way a car works. In a car, dirty oil clogs filters, impairing the function of the motor. If the oil were never changed, the car would eventually grind to a halt. When blood lacks oxygen and is polluted with chemicals and impurities, a similar breakdown may be expected in the body. If you owned a very expensive car, would you run it on the cheapest gasoline?

The simplest and most effective treatment for cleansing the blood is aloe vera. Aloe vera is a powerful antioxidant that brings oxygen to every cell in the body. By cleansing the kidneys, it rids the body of toxic wastes and aids digestion. (It is also a mild, natural laxative.) It increases circulation and relieves constipation. There is more information about the healing properties of aloe vera in Chapter 5.

In a detoxification program, drink two to four ounces of aloe vera juice in an eight-ounce glass of water or fruit juice twice a day, at the time of your choice, for three to four weeks. (Any brand of 100 percent pure aloe vera juice will do. It should be available at your local health food store.) This may be repeated as often as you feel necessary. If your diet is free of any "pollutants," such as sugar, alcohol, artificial colorings, preservatives, etc., you may need to cleanse the blood only two or three times a year. If, like most of us, your diet wavers a bit, you may want to repeat this cleansing every other month. Some people include two ounces of aloe vera juice daily in their diet as a preventative against toxicity. If you do this, extra cleansing may be unnecessary.

Another gentle type of cleansing may be obtained by ingesting a variety of herbs that are available in natural food stores. Black walnut leaf tea is a favorite of mine.

Reducing Water Retention

When the body is retaining water, there is a lack of balance—too high a concentration of something, usually sodium (salt) or protein, which the body tries to compensate for by diluting it with water. Too much salt results in a lack of potassium, which regulates the water balance in cells. One way to avoid water retention is to cut down on the amount of salt in your diet, as suggested above.

Although many doctors prescribe diuretic pills as a cure for water retention, these substances can add to the core of the problem by robbing the body of potassium. A sufficient daily intake of potassium will help your body maintain an even water level balance in the cells. All fruits and vegetables contain potassium; however, some contain more than others. Bananas, dark green leafy vegetables, dried apricots, potatoes (including the skin), dairy products, whole grains, dried beans, sunflower seeds, and garbanzo beans are excellent sources of potassium.

Remember to drink lots of good water and herbal teas too. If you don't drink a sufficient amount of water, your body will retain the water it has, acting as if there is a shortage. Drinking six glasses of sodium-free water daily helps to flush toxins from your body and keep the water level in your cells balanced.

A good detoxification diet consists of simply eating fresh fruits and juices, vegetables, and brown rice for several days. You can add to this regimen protein powder drinks and any number of detoxifying herbal teas. Once again, I recommend perusing the bookshelves of your local natural food store for books on this subject. There are dozens of different detoxification eating plans, some specially designed to treat specific toxic symptoms.

Once you become aware of how good your body feels when it is "clean," you will be able to distinguish the substances that make you feel sluggish or are a drain on your energy.

5 Super Supplements: Anti-Aging Nutrients

The more closely you follow my 10 Basic Rules for Anti-Aging Eating (Chapter 4), the more likely that you will meet your nutritional needs. But unless you get all of your fruits and vegetables on a seasonal basis from organic sources, you may not get all of the vitamins and minerals you personally need. Also, if you indulge in any of the substances that cause depletion (caffeine, cigarettes, alcohol, artificial coloring, artificial flavoring, nitrites, nitrates, preservatives, aspirin, recreational drugs, birth-control pills, antibiotics), or if you live in a smoggy area, you will absolutely need to augment your diet with supplemental vitamins and minerals.

There are dozens of multiple vitamin/mineral combinations on the market today, and it can be very confusing to determine how much of what you should be taking. You can be certain, however, that the one-capsule-a-day variety will probably not meet your needs. You should consider formulas with several tablets taken daily in order to get adequate amounts of minerals, antioxidants, and trace elements. A number of products have been formulated specifically for women, offering help with PMS symptoms and other female needs. Usually, someone at your local health food store can help you choose a formula, or you might consult with a nutritionist about what is right for you.

Antioxidant Skin Supplements

In Chapters 1 and 3, I discussed the role of free radicals in the aging process. As noted, free radicals are unstable oxygen molecules that attach themselves to other molecules, attacking cell membranes and vital cell components. They can deactivate important enzymes and even damage DNA. The oxidation process that takes place is believed to be responsible for the breakdown of cells that precedes aging and disease.

The "father" of the free-radical theory of aging, Dr. Denhan Harman of the University of Nebraska, discovered the existence of free radicals during longevity experiments with rodents. To counteract the effect, Dr. Harman fed the test animals a diet high in the antioxidant preservatives BHT and MEA. He was able to extend their life spans by as much as 29 percent. I do not, however, recommend ingesting a diet high in artificial preservatives. For human beings, there is a healthier way to accomplish a similar result—through the use of vitamins.

Antioxidant vitamins and nutrients work to "sweep up" free radicals and neutralize them. These vitamins have been touted by nutritionists and "health nuts" for years as being useful for prolonging sex drive, increasing energy, protecting against sickness, preventing cancer and arteriosclerosis, and contributing to longevity. The primary antioxidant supplements are vitamin A in the form of beta-carotene, vitamins C and E, and the trace elements selenium and zinc, but there are also a number of other antioxidant nutrients.

Vitamin E

Vitamin E is the main fat-soluble antioxidant used in the body. Fat-soluble means that a substance must be taken with foods containing fat in order to be assimilated. Vitamin E has the strongest healing ability of all the vitamins. It helps protect both vitamin A and other oils or fats from oxidation (becoming rancid), and it transports oxygen to cells. Known also as tocopherol, vitamin E establishes itself in cell membranes and protects against free-radical attack.

Although vitamin E is crucial to body health, it is not manufactured by the body. To receive the antioxidant effects of vitamin E, you will need to take more than the current RDA (recommended daily allowance). I prescribe a supplemental dosage ranging from 800 to 1200 I.U. (international units) a day. You can split the dosage into two smaller ones, both taken with meals containing fat. Along with that, take vitamin A and zinc. Be sure you get vitamin E in the form of natural d-Alpha tocopherol rather than dl-Alpha tocopherol, which is cheaper but has half the potency. Food sources of vitamin E include legumes, fresh vegetables, wheat-germ oil, raw wheat germ, almonds, pecans, hazelnuts, sunflower seeds, and oils made from sesame seeds, sunflower seeds, canola, soy, and corn.

Vitamin E may also be applied directly to the skin via lotions and creams, as it is a highly moisturizing oil. Applied topically, it has a number of benefits, including protection from ultraviolet light, reducing the appearance of fine lines and wrinkles, and helping to delay the progression of aging. Taken internally or externally, it helps heal scarring and wounds. However, if you've ever used vitamin E oil on the skin, you'll know that it is very thick and heavy, making it difficult to wear on the face during the day. It's easiest to use as a treatment, left on the skin for several hours then washed off.

Vitamin C

As well as protecting the body in many ways, vitamin C is also an excellent antioxidant. Along with vitamin E, it helps prevent LDL cholesterol from being oxidized into its damaging form. It is important in the metabolism of amino acids, and it activates folic acid and prevents the oxidation of other vitamins.

With regard to the skin, vitamin C helps the body heal itself, resist infection, form pigment, and build and maintain collagen and elastin. Because of its importance to these functions, our need for vitamin C increases with age. It strengthens the skin, and when taken with rutin (a naturally occurring form of vitamin C derived from either eucalyptus or eucommia leaves), it will also strengthen capillary walls. This means lower susceptibility to broken capillaries. Vitamin C is greatly depleted by smoking (one cigarette uses up 25 milligrams), and by caffeine, alcohol, aspirin, recreational drugs, and estrogen drugs.

While the RDA for vitamin C is only 60 milligrams a day, multigram amounts (1000 to 4000 milligrams) can be taken without harmful side effects. High doses can cause stomach upset for some people, so it's a good idea to build up slowly from 500 milligrams three times a day. You may also want to try a buffered source, which is easier on the stomach. I recommend taking 2 to 4 grams (2000 to 4000 milligrams) a day throughout the day, with food. If taking more than 1000 milligrams, split the dosage into two or three smaller doses taken during the course of the day, with or without meals. Take with bioflavonoids (sometimes called vitamin P), vitamin D, and rutin to strengthen thin, sensitive skin.

Fruits such as citrus, papaya, strawberries, and cantaloupe are high in vitamin C, as are dark green vegetables, yellow vegetables, cabbage, potatoes, and rose hips.

Beta-Carotene and Vitamin A

Beta-carotene and vitamin A are both powerful antioxidants. Beta-carotene is a highly effective anti-infective that is converted by the liver into vitamin A as it is needed. Beta-carotene is found in any fruit or vegetable that is green, yellow, orange, or red. We are hearing more and more about beta-carotene these days because of studies that have shown it to be effective in preventing cancers of various kinds.

Vitamin A is a fat-soluble vitamin derived from animal sources, primarily dairy products and fish. As well as being crucial to eyesight and the production of new cells, vitamin

A is needed for the health and repair of mucous membranes—keeping the digestive tract and the vagina moist. Vitamin A is also important for hormonal balance and for the conversion of cholesterol into adrenal hormones. It is easily depleted by stress and illness. Without sufficient vitamin A, the body will deplete itself of vitamin C.

Vitamin A is one of the two vitamins that can be absorbed by the skin, and it is highly beneficial to hair, skin, and nails. It helps to fight acne and premenstrual skin eruptions. Vitamin A acid, a metabolite of vitamin A that is readily absorbed through the skin, increases blood flow, stimulates the skin, and helps to keep it supple. Experiments conducted by Herman Pinkus, M.D., and Rose Hunter proved that "vitamin A has an 'antikeratinizing' effect that is achieved by cells remaining immature (young) longer." Dermatologist Dr. Albert Kligman, the inventor of Retin-A, says that vitamin A now is being used in tumor therapy and in preventing postsurgical cancer recurrences. It may also prevent precancerous skin tumors.

Vitamin A is the only vitamin that is stored by the body, making it potentially toxic if too much is stored. Overdoses of vitamin A can cause headaches, liver damage, and other serious symptoms. That is why it is safer to take large doses as beta-carotene. Supplemental beta-carotene can be taken in dosages that range from 5000 to 25,000 I.U. daily.

Selenium

Selenium is a trace mineral that can be toxic in large doses but is important in very small doses (30 to 200 micrograms daily). A powerful antioxidant, it is considered an immune-system stimulant and is especially important in preventing cancer. Selenium works with vitamin E to prevent the accumulation of cholesterol in the blood and to protect against heart disease. With regard to the skin, selenium enhances elasticity. The most effective sources of selenium are garlic (personally, I suspect that this is why

Italians have such exquisite skin), brewer's yeast, sesame seeds, kelp, tuna, oysters, fish, and organ meats. It is also found in meat, grains, and dairy products.

Zinc

Zinc is another crucial antioxidant trace mineral. It is essential to the formation of insulin, to immune-system strength, and to the health of glandular, sexual, and reproductive systems. Zinc is very important for healthy skin and necessary for collagen formation. It aids in the assimilation of vitamins A and B and combines with vitamin A for protein synthesis, which makes healing possible. Zinc helps to prevent acne, regulate oil glands, and clear problem skin. Good sources of zinc are eggs, fish, peas, nuts, beans, grains, brewer's yeast, sunflower seeds, dairy products, and mushrooms. For supplemental zinc, I recommend taking 15 to 30 milligrams once daily with food. When you first begin taking zinc, it can cause slight nausea, so build up to the recommended dosage slowly over a period of two weeks and always take it with food.

There are a number of other antioxidants that may be formulated along with the ones listed above. These include the enzymes CoQ-10, superoxide dismutase (SOD), and glutathione perioxidase, which are found in many good antioxidant supplement products.

Vitamin B Complex

Other vitamins that are not antioxidants but are crucial to general health as well as skin health are the B vitamins, sometimes referred to as B complex because they are 11 vitamins taken in combination. They are water-soluble and not stored by the body. Vital for building protein, they are responsible for cell generation and repair. Like natural tranquilizers, they help to keep the nervous system healthy and are known as the "antistress" vitamins. Vitamin B also helps the liver make glycogen, which enables the skin to rid itself of dead cells. B complex is greatly depleted by smoking, alcohol, recreational drugs, sunning, oral contraceptives, and estrogen drugs.

I recommend a B complex that has 100 milligrams of B_1, B_2, B_6, and B_{12} plus at least 400 milligrams of B_3 and B_5, as well as PABA, niacin, pantothenic acid, choline, inositol, and biotin. During times of stress the dosage may be doubled. It may be split into two doses, to be taken with meals, preferably in the morning and afternoon. Sources of B vitamins include whole-grain products, bananas, eggs, nuts, seeds, chicken, fish, shellfish, mushrooms, potatoes, legumes, yogurt, cheese, and brewer's yeast. *NOTE:* Liver is very high in B vitamins, but because its role is to filter toxins, I do not recommend eating it. If you love it, choose only liver from organically raised, free-range cattle or chickens.

Anti-Aging Aloe Vera

One of the most valuable supplements for natural anti-aging is the juice of the aloe vera plant. Applied externally, it can do wonders for the skin, but it can also be taken internally to cleanse the body.

I discovered aloe vera 25 years ago on a trip to Hawaii. A friend recommended I rub some of the plant's jellylike substance on my badly sunburned skin. Not only did it soothe the pain, but by the next morning the redness had turned into a golden tan. Since then, aloe vera has become central to my skin-care system, and I have continued to discover more and more of its benefits. Of course, I am not the first to do so: Aloe vera is one of the oldest medicinal plants known to humankind. It was used by the ancient Egyptians, who considered it sacred because of its miraculous healing powers. There are references to aloe in the Bible, and it was used during the Roman Empire. Native Americans of the West used it for healing and as a cosmetic.

Aloe vera contains the key trace minerals calcium, potassium, sodium, choline, manganese, magnesium, zinc, copper, and chromium, and the vitamins B_1, B_2, niacinamide, and B_6, all of which are crucial to our health. Because of its antimicrobial effects, aloe is a natural antiseptic that helps to fight infection. Experiments by Dr. Wendell D. Winters, professor of microbiology at the University of Texas, San Antonio, proved that fresh aloe extract promotes healing in a fashion similar to the body's own response.

My personal experience has been with the power of aloe to repair and rejuvenate damaged skin when products containing aloe vera are used on a daily basis. Over the years, I've seen amazing results for all types of skin. People with dry skin noticed that their skin became less dry or, in some cases, no longer dry. People with combination skin found that their skin became more balanced—the oily areas less oily, the dry areas less dry. Breakouts, which can be common in oily areas, either lessened or ceased completely. A definite tightening effect could be felt and seen, and pores appeared to become smaller. For those with oily skin, there was a marked decrease in the amount of oil on the skin, and a lessening or ceasing of oil-related blemishes. The "shine" stayed away longer, makeup stayed on better, and skin tone improved.

Possibly the most dramatic differences were noticed by people with acne. Two tablespoons of the pure gel were applied to the affected areas and allowed to dry. This had an immediate calming effect on skin, lessening redness and discomfort. Applications three times a day helped to kill bacteria and heal blemishes two to three times faster than normal. The overall look of the complexion was greatly improved. Continued use over several months brought even greater improvement. However, because of its astringent effect, aloe vera causes dryness when used on a regular basis in its pure form. For this reason, I always recommend using an aloe-rich product on a daily basis and using the pure form for medicinal treatment only.

One of the most unique qualities of aloe vera may be its penetrating ability: It goes into the skin to the water-retaining level. This means your skin receives all of the good vitamins and minerals aloe contains *where it can use them*. A natural oxygenator, aloe helps skin attract and hold oxygen. When the skin is holding oxygen, it is holding moisture—perhaps the most beneficial function of any cosmetic. Like papayas, pineapples, and alphahydroxy acids, aloe vera contains enzymes that help to break down dead cells on the skin's surface.

In summary, aloe vera is beneficial to skin in the following ways:

◆ It penetrates deeply, carrying nutrients and oxygen.

◆ Its enzymes dissolve dead surface-layer cells.

◆ It helps the skin hold moisture.

◆ It balances the skin's pH.

◆ It tightens pores.

◆ Its antibacterial qualities fight infection.

All of these effects translate into smoother skin, good skin tone, fewer lines, less dryness and oiliness, and fewer breakouts.

When using aloe on the skin, follow these guidelines:

◆ It is best to use a formulated aloe vera product (with aloe as a primary ingredient) rather than pure aloe gels and juices. These usually contain potassium sorbate or sorbic acid as preservatives, making them irritating to some people. Although some people are not affected at all by these additives, others experience redness and/or a burning sensation that lasts from 10 to 45 minutes.

◆ People with dry skin should only use a water-diluted three-to-one mixture of the juice (three parts water to one part aloe vera).

◆ People with oily skin may use a very mild astringent made of equal parts of aloe vera gel or juice, witch hazel, and water. Adding a small amount of alum to the mixture gives it more of a drying effect (one-half teaspoon of alum to eight ounces of an aloe–witch hazel mixture).

◆ Aloe vera extract combined with seaweed extract makes the most effective toner I have ever found. It tightens the skin, adjusts the pH, attracts oxygen, and really penetrates.

◆ Applying moisturizer to the skin while it is still damp with an aloe toner boosts the function of the moisturizer and helps it to penetrate.

◆ Applying makeup over an aloe vera toner helps it to last longer and look smoother.

Taking Aloe Vera Internally

Aloe vera juice may also be taken internally. Its unique cleansing qualities purify the blood, kidneys, and intestines, and carry oxygen and nutrients including the antioxidant vitamins A, C, and niacinamide. For people with acne or excessively dry skin, it is especially beneficial if taken regularly over several months. I recommend drinking aloe vera juice for cleansing the blood in a program of detoxification according to these guidelines:

◆ *For general health:* two ounces in a large glass of water once a day, three to seven times a week.

◆ *For constipation and/or detoxification:* three to four ounces in a large glass of water two times a day for two days, then once a day for two weeks.

◆ *For dry skin:* two ounces in a large glass of water every day until condition improves, then decrease to three times a week.

◆ *For acne:* three ounces in a large glass of water three times a day for 10 days, then decrease to two ounces twice a day for a month. Continue this dosage until the condition greatly improves, then cut down to one ounce twice a day until the condition is cleared. It is a good idea to continue drinking small amounts of aloe a few times a week to help prevent acne flare-ups.

Aloe vera is available in most health food stores as either juice or gel. Any brand that is between 98 and 100 percent pure aloe and does not contain either potassium sorbate or sorbic acid is recommended. In my extensive research into the latest experiments in the United States, I have found no record of adverse reaction to aloe vera. It has been shown to be beneficial to everyone, regardless of age. However, I caution anyone with a history of serious medical problems or allergies to check with her doctor before beginning any self-prescribed program.

In addition to the vitamins and supplements I have described here, there are many others that can be very valuable both in healing specific problems and promoting general health. Some health practitioners and longevity enthusiasts strongly recommend taking supplemental amino acids, the building blocks of proteins; many nutritionists and herbal specialists promote the use of herbs and herbal products. Personally, I have benefited greatly from the use of both amino acids and herbs, but I am not qualified to recommend specific supplements. The information could easily fill another book this size, and there are already a number of very good books on herbal remedies. Take the time to browse through a health-oriented bookstore or your local library for books on herbs and refer to the Recommended Reading list at the end of this book. Once you've read a book about herbs, you'll probably want to know more—with herbs, the possibilities are endless!

6

Fabulously Fit: Reducing Stress with Exercise

If you want to look younger and live a longer, healthier, happier life, the way you use your body—keeping it fit—is as important as what you feed it. This chapter is about the amazing benefits of exercise and also about ways to reduce the stress in your life. I've put these two topics together because they are very much related. The number-one most effective stress reducer is regular exercise. Exercise is also crucial to your overall health as well as beneficial to your skin.

The Benefits of Exercise

Recent research into longevity has proven the commonsense notion that active people live longer and are healthier than sedentary ones. The good news about exercise is that it does not have to be strenuous to effectively improve cardiovascular function. Studies have shown that people who walk briskly for half an hour six days a week have similar mortality rates to those who run 40 or 50 miles a week. Of course, the runner will be more physically fit, but in terms of maintaining overall body health, regular mild activity does the job. There is evidence that regular workouts slow down the stiffening of arteries (the result of thickening arterial walls) and that strenuous workouts can reverse any clogging of arteries present in those with coronary disease.

The most important aspect of exercise is consistency. "Vegging out" during the week and then doing a couple of aerobics classes on the weekend can be very stressful to the body, not to mention causing sore, aching muscles. Far better are regular, shorter exercise sessions. For optimum results, most experts recommend daily exercise, but if this is not possible, the next best is exercising at least three times a week. If your goal is to keep your body looking young as well as remaining healthy, a muscle-toning and -building program will also be required.

I have always recommended finding several types of exercise you really enjoy doing and varying them throughout the week. Recently, this type of diversified exercise program has been given the name "cross training." Its benefits are many: There is no exercise burnout; all parts of your body are exercised; and you develop a variety of skills, which is good for your psyche as well as your body. You can also change your exercise routine seasonally, enjoying cross-country skiing and skating in winter, rollerblading, hiking, and swimming in the summer.

Exercise is one of the prime ways to control weight and maintain a trim, shapely body. It's also necessary for promoting cardiovascular health and preventing heart disease. But exercise is equally beneficial to the skin. A daily routine of some type of aerobic activity helps the skin stay young by

◆ increasing circulation, bringing nutrients to cells and organs;

◆ revving up oil- and sweat-gland production to combat the "slowdown" of aging skin;

◆ increasing oxygen intake, which aids the production of new cells;

◆ helping to rid the body of toxins that can cause breakouts and unhealthy skin; and

◆ boosting collagen and elastin production to strengthen connective tissue and maintain elasticity.

This last benefit deserves some explanation. Prolonged, vigorous exercise raises the temperature of the skin, which causes it to produce more collagen. In his book *Jump for Joy*, James White, Ph.D., an exercise physiologist at the University of California, San Diego, states, "The cells in the base layer of skin, where skin cells are formed, actually become more active with exercise. More of the chemical substances that are used to produce the elastic fibers (collagen and elastin) can be found in the cells of people who exercise." Dr. White used three-dimensional photos to measure number, depth, width, and distribution of wrinkles in groups of women. He found that those who either worked out indoors or ran while using a sunblock, for 30 to 40 minutes daily, had fewer wrinkles than nonexercisers; bags under the eyes also disappeared.

"But I'm too old to start exercising now!" you say. Not true! Some of the most encouraging research in aging today reveals that it is never too late to take up some form of exercise. The benefits of physical activity are as great for a 90-year-old as for a 20-year-old. Even someone who has always been sedentary will improve his or her health almost immediately upon beginning an exercise program.

If you want to lose weight and keep it off, increasing your exercise should go hand in hand with a sensible way of eating. Exercise raises your metabolism, which means that you will burn calories faster and more effectively.

You don't have to start lifting weights or running marathons. Any kind of regular physical activity that gets your heart pumping faster and your muscles moving is valuable. Start slowly, and build as you begin to feel stronger and see good results. The more active you become, the more activity you'll crave because exercise is addictive, just like chocolate, and for the same reason. Both stimulate the body to produce beta-endorphin, a hormone that acts as a mood elevator (antidepressant) and an appetite suppressant. Researchers believe it to be the same hormone that is released when you're in love. I don't think anything could feel better than that!

The Stress Connection

Those same beta-endorphins that are increased with exercise are reduced with stress. The body's reaction to stressful situations is the "fight-or-flight" mechanism in which our normal anabolic metabolism converts to a catabolic metabolism, in which the body breaks down its own tissues. The adrenaline produced under stress causes a variety of stress reactions—rapid breathing, muscular tension, and rising blood pressure as well as the suppression of digestion, hunger, and sexual desire.

The level of endorphins, the body's natural tranquilizers, falls as a result of stress. In an effort to make you feel better, the body releases pain-relieving substances that interfere with intestinal secretions necessary for digestion. For this reason, stress is often associated with indigestion. To make matters worse, stress produces a rise in the blood level of free fatty acids, organic acids that combine with glycerin to form fat. This explains the stress-related rise in blood cholesterol levels. Triglycerides, the type of fat stored by the body and linked to heart disease, also increase by as much as 50 percent. Most of us are also aware of the impact of stress on the skin: Think about when you've had facial breakouts—usually when you menstruate, ovulate, or are very nervous or stressed.

The fight-or-flight mechanism of stress response is vital in some situations, but if stress continues over a prolonged period of time, the catabolic metabolism damages the body, resulting in such specific problems as hypertension, ulcers, colitis, and psoriasis. Stress seems to get blamed for most everything in our society now, from job burnout to heart disease. But what we may not realize is that stress is one of the major causes of aging. Prolonged stress also works over time to weaken the entire immune system, resulting in fatigue, depression, and illness. Many of these problems are characteristic of aging. Also, the older we get, the less easily we recover from stressful situations.

Types of Stress

There are actually two types of stress—what might be called good stress and bad stress. "Bad" stress is distress; it occurs when we are having real problems at home or work that are physically, emotionally, or mentally trying. We often feel out of control, angry, afraid, or hopeless. "Good" stress is more like a challenging situation—when we are making changes in our lives, growing in new areas, or taking on new responsibilities that will ultimately enrich us. A promotion can be stressful, as can having a new baby or a new romance. This type of stress can become distress if we let it, if we let ourselves become overwhelmed and lose perspective.

It is not merely the stressful occurrence that affects us, it is our *perception* of the occurrence. What is stressful to one person may not be to another—it depends on how an event or situation is interpreted. Worry, which generally follows a stressful occurrence, perpetuates the stress effect. How you deal with the *aftermath* of a stressful situation is what really makes the difference. Learning how to counter these effects can not only add years to your life, it will also make daily living more pleasant. When you feel better, your body functions better and ultimately looks better.

Basically, when we are under stress, we first try to compensate by doing more—working harder, trying new things. When the stress continues and overproducing doesn't work, we tend to just give up. This same process occurs in a body under stress. It starts overproducing also, trying harder to give us signals that what we are doing isn't working. You know the signs: the headache, the aching back, the indigestion, the inability to sleep. In order to keep ourselves going, we take a couple of aspirin, drink some coffee, or eat a chocolate bar. Instead, we could prevent stress from building up by paying attention to our body signals and giving ourselves what we really need. We might take a short nap instead of the coffee, do some yoga to stretch our shoulders and back, do a bit of slow, deep breathing, or just sit for a few moments and look out the window and drink a cup of herbal tea.

Stress can also be caused by situations outside ourselves—the uncomfortable, unhealthy, or hostile aspects of our environment, such as air pollution from smog or cigarettes, excessive heat or cold, conditioned air that lacks humidity, fluorescent lights, traveling, or even sleeping in an uncomfortable bed. It's not possible these days to avoid all stressful situations; there is too much in modern life that is simply unavoidable. But you can prepare your body and mind for stress so that you're able to reduce its negative effects. Even if the best you can do is shorten the amount of time you feel stressed, you'll be accomplishing a great deal.

It is also important to keep your body physically primed for dealing with stress. Substances such as caffeine, tobacco, and white sugar rob the body of the nutrients necessary to maintain body–mind balance, specifically vitamins A, B complex, E, and C; oxygen; minerals; and trace elements. Caffeine and tobacco also cause constriction of blood vessels and capillaries that carry nutrients to cells. When you're under stress, you should take vitamin B complex (100 milligrams two times daily) and calcium and magnesium (1000 milligrams two times a day and before bed). Some calcium supplements are not digested by the body. To test yours, put a tablet in some distilled white vinegar; if it has not dissolved in an hour, it will not dissolve in your stomach.

To relax in stressful situations, rather than taking drugs like alcohol or Valium, you may want to try some herbal and naturopathic alternatives. Valerian root is a natural muscle relaxant that helps you sleep, and passionflower is also relaxing. A number of herbs used for centuries by herbalists have recently been shown to increase the body's ability to withstand stress. They are known as "adaptogens" and include ginseng, dong quai, gotu kola, watercress, sumac, lavender, and aloe vera. What these herbs have in common is a substance called germanium, a trace mineral like selenium that helps to neutralize free radicals and also works to help the body use oxygen more efficiently. Homeopathic relaxation products include Calmes, Nervosan, and the Bach flower remedies.

Another problem with stress is that it affects the way you eat. When we are very busy during the day, we are more likely to grab a fast-food hamburger or perhaps a couple of chocolate bars. The solution is to plan ahead. On days when you know you're going to be very busy or dealing with stressful situations, plan what you're going to eat. Rather than grabbing food on the run, take a supply of nutrient-rich food with you and eat some every two to three hours. Snacks like fat-free yogurt, pretzels, fat-free tortilla chips, air-popped popcorn, fresh or dried fruit, a tuna sandwich, and a bottle of water can get you through some rough spots in the day without having to revert to coffee and doughnuts.

Reducing Stress Through Exercise

Once you know you're stressed out, there are a number of ways to disconnect and recover, but probably the most effective one is exercise. As discussed above, exercise is not only good for your health and longevity, it also makes you feel better. Those beta-endorphins created by aerobic activity will help calm stress reactions.

Exercise is truly a holistic therapy because it benefits the body in virtually every way—internally, externally, and mentally. Any technique that effectively counters stress is good for mental health, physical health, and the health of the skin. Exercise also works to build self-esteem. Who doesn't feel good about themselves when they've taken a long walk or had a vigorous workout? Many of us do our best problem-solving while exercising. Running, walking, swimming, biking, or any repetitive movement can become a kind of meditation that helps focus the mind as well as soothe the soul.

An extra bonus may be that exercise also prepares us for handling unexpected stress better than those who don't exercise. New research by Drs. Diane and Robert Hales has shown this to be true. They explain it this way: "Aerobic exercise can cause physical symptoms similar to a stressful situation, though not as intense . . . the racing heart, higher blood pressure, etc. In this way, intense workouts 'condition' your body to cope with stress when you're in a sudden jam."

You can get the same kind of stress reduction with anaerobic exercise such as yoga. Yoga is based on the premise that the vital energy that is stored in the body may be released and used to overcome deterioration of the body and mind. There are several types of yoga that are now taught nationwide, and they vary greatly in terms of their approach to stretching. Hatha yoga incorporates slow, stretching movements to tone the muscles, and deep breathing to bring oxygen to the blood and to soothe the mind. This is an excellent form of exercise for people who find it hard to relax. Because of its gentleness and slowness, it is also excellent for older people whose movements may be impaired. The Iyengar version of hatha yoga features more challenging positions and also tones the muscles. Ashtanga yoga is a different form of yoga, sometimes referred to as "aerobic or macho yoga," as it gives you quite a physical workout. It involves relatively fast movement through the various positions and intense breathing patterns. Beware, however, because Ashtanga yoga is very difficult and is appropriate for the athletic only.

Yoga videotapes are a great way to try the different types and styles of yoga before seeking out a class. Often, you can borrow them from your public library. There are a number of yoga videotapes on the market that I have listed at the end of this book.

One of my favorite forms of exercise, especially if you dislike aerobics and are not athletically inclined, is Callanetics. This gentle yet effective program combines isometrics (repetitive movements of one muscle at a time in a very small motion) with stretching exercises. Pursued diligently, it can rid the body of saddlebags and bulges faster than any other type of exercise I know. It can be practiced using the book or the videotapes. The tapes are easy to follow, and offer a good variety of exercises from beginning to advanced.

Improving the Quality of Your Sleep

Also crucial to recovering from stress is a good night's sleep. There are several things you can do to help you get to sleep and to ensure that your sleep is restful.

1. Meditate before bedtime, either by a method you have learned or with one of the many meditation audiotapes available.

2. Make a list of all the things that could occupy your mind and prevent you from "shutting down" for the night. This will keep you from lying awake in bed reviewing what didn't get done or what needs to be done. Making the list will free your mind to turn off once you get into bed.

3. Drink a cup of warm skim milk. The calcium and tryptophane will help you relax and fall asleep.

4. Try one of the herbal sleep combinations sold in natural food stores.

5. *Love your bed!* Be sure that your mattress, pillows, sheets, and blankets are comfortable and comforting to you. If you tend to be cold, invest in a down comforter. The natural insulating quality of down keeps

you warmer than any blanket, allowing you to relax rather than huddling to keep warm.

You should also be aware of how you sleep. If you wake up looking wrinkled and haggard after sleeping, you may be creating lines and wrinkles by pressing them into your face with pillows and bedding. The best way to sleep is on your back with your head slightly elevated. Some people prefer sleeping pillowless, but this causes fluids to drain downward, toward the top of the head, resulting in puffiness around the eyes. Conversely, sleeping with the head too propped up can cause wrinkling of the front of the neck.

The right kind of pillow can help you sleep on your back. Try the classic Japanese pillow, which consists of a hard roll of cotton batting that goes under your neck, or a foam pillow shaped like a rectangle with a U cut into one side. This supports the neck and shoulders very comfortably and doesn't allow your body to roll over easily. The angle of the head is good, and no additional pillow is necessary. There is also a newly designed foam rubber pillow that lets you sleep on your side without mashing your face. Its center is scooped out, yet it supports the top of the head, neck, and chin. You can find these pillows in SelfCare Catalogue (1-800-345-3371), as well as in the mail-order section of health magazines.

Another helpful hint for teaching yourself to sleep on your back is to use a simple deep relaxation technique while falling asleep. Lie on your back with feet comfortably apart and with arms alongside your body but not touching it. Take three deep breaths, inhaling slowly through the nose; hold for a few seconds, then exhale slowly through the nose. Focus your attention on the tips of your toes for a few seconds, telling yourself that they are relaxed. Slowly move up your body, by three- to five-inch intervals—toes to ankles to shins to calves to knees, and so on—pausing at each spot for 1 to 20 seconds and telling yourself that that spot is relaxed. I usually don't get any farther than my navel before I'm asleep. It's amazing how relaxing this is.

It may take awhile before you can sleep an entire night on your back, but even if you manage only half a night, it will be an improvement.

Taking Time to Nurture Yourself

We are often so busy expending energy—giving it to our work, our families, our relationships—we forget that we need to take energy in. Part of recharging is relaxing (you can't take energy in unless you are open to it), but relaxing doesn't necessarily mean doing nothing. Recharging comes from nurturing ourselves—asking ourselves what we *really* need and giving it to ourselves. How we recharge may be a personal preference: Some of us like to be alone, whereas others like hanging out with friends. I love to dance or hike. If I'm in a quiet mood I paint or read. You might like to sit and listen to your favorite music. You may have a hobby that relaxes you, or you may find that watching a movie gives you the break you need.

I have always found water to be a relaxing element—simply taking a long bath or a shower, or floating in a pool or the ocean. Saunas, steam rooms, and hot tubs are particularly wonderful ways to relax. I find a 10-minute steam to be the fastest way to unwind. There is something almost magical about being warm and wet simultaneously—perhaps because it duplicates the experience of being in the womb. Whatever it is, it really works for me!

However, as good as hydrotherapy is for your frame of mind, it can be damaging to your skin. If you're going to get wet, a few preventive measures will allow you to get maximum relaxation with no harm. Always cleanse your face before any of these treatments. In saunas and steam rooms, protect delicate skin on the face with a wet towel or cloth and never stay in for more than 10 minutes at a time. Turn saunas into steams by putting water on the rocks; in dry saunas, it takes most women too long to perspire, and the dry heat can break capillaries. In hot tubs, don't dunk your face under the water or even splash this water on your face, as the chlorine and bromine are too harsh. Always take a cold shower to close down pores immediately afterward. Be sure to wash toxins from your skin with a gentle body cleanser, and use a body moisturizer.

For many people, meditation is the ultimate form of relaxation, stress reduction, and self-nurturing. It can also be a path to self-knowledge and enlightenment. If you are interested in spiritual growth and development through meditation, you may want to find a teacher or group that can guide you on the path. If you want to relax and clear your mind, you can try any number of simple meditation techniques, such as repeating a mantra (a sound or word), counting your breaths, or simply paying attention to your breathing.

Of course, "simply paying attention to your breathing" is probably one of the most difficult things a human being can do. You will find that the mind is a very busy little monkey indeed, and that after a few conscious breaths you are lost in thought once again. Observing yourself gaining and losing awareness *is* the process of meditation. A meditative state is not something you can "achieve" quickly or easily; it takes patience and perseverance. In fact, developing those two skills is part of the process of learning meditation. You may want to experiment with different types of meditation to find the form that works best for you. Try some of the many audio tapes available to get a first-hand experience of different types of meditation.

Even if you don't formally meditate, you can take time during each day just to close your eyes and focus on your breathing, inhaling and exhaling several deep breaths through your nose. Roll and shrug your shoulders to loosen the tension there. If you are at a desk, get up and walk around frequently, and don't forget to drink your six glasses of water. That will not only flush your body, it will make sure you get up often to go to the bathroom!

Another way we nurture ourselves is getting out into nature, away from the noise and stimulus of our daily lives.

Eat lunch in the park, take a walk after work, watch the sunset, or go outside at night to contemplate the stars.

And don't forget what is probably the all-time best stress reducer—laughter. Find someone or something to make you laugh, and you'll shed stress instantly.

Whatever way you choose to nurture yourself, the important thing to remember is to do it often.

7 Nonsurgical Face Treatments for Damaged Skin

Now you know how to keep your skin healthy through diet, supplements, exercise, and stress reduction, but what can you do about skin that has already suffered the ravages of time? What can be done about the damage from years of careless sunning, furrowed brows, or bouts with acne? Are there natural anti-aging treatments for those of you with deep wrinkles, splotchy skin, age spots, and acne scars, or is cosmetic surgery the only answer to looking great as we get older?

While I am not opposed to cosmetic surgery when it is appropriate, I believe there are a number of effective treatments for damaged skin that lessen the appearance of aging without resorting to expensive and invasive surgery. Before we look at these natural alternatives, I'll briefly discuss cosmetic surgery (sometimes called plastic surgery).

Concerning Cosmetic Surgery

Cosmetic surgery can be a very effective, appropriate treatment under the right circumstances and for the right reasons. In some instances, it may not only improve appearances, it can also change lives. Over the years, I have met many people who rave about the results their surgery produced and how happy it has made them.

In the course of my research into cosmetic surgery, I have viewed hundreds of "before" and "after" photographs of women who have undergone plastic surgery. I have seen pictures of nose jobs, eye-lifts, brow-lifts, chin and cheek-bone implantations, liposuction, and full face-lifts. The "before" photographs showed women whose degenerated skin condition (wrinkles, jowls, double chins, sagging necks, drooping eyes) made them look as much as 20 years older than they were. The state of mind that came through these pictures to me was nothing short of despair. Many women looked as if their lives were over, and some were only in their fifties. While viewing the "after" pictures of the same women, the thing that impressed me most, aside from the incredible visual results, was the feeling of aliveness that was communicated. Now these faces looked truly happy. Any remaining doubts I had as to the necessity or usefulness of cosmetic surgery were completely dispelled.

If you feel that cosmetic surgery is right for you, let me give you just two pieces of very important advice. First, look carefully at your motives for wanting surgery, and make sure that surgery is really going to get you the results you seek. For example, if what you want is "to feel sexier," liposuction may not be the appropriate route. There may be other ways to accomplish the same thing, like losing some weight, sculpting your body with exercise, or getting some therapy for emotional issues. Make sure the operation you want will achieve the results you want, and be sure to consider all of the alternatives.

Second, be very careful in choosing your cosmetic surgeon. Take as much time as you need to feel absolutely sure that you have made the correct choice. To find the doctor right for you, ask your family physician for some recommendations, inquire at local medical schools or hospitals, or call the American Society of Plastic and Reconstructive Surgeons or the American Academy of Cosmetic Surgery for information and recommendations. Then talk to people you know who have been through surgery, or, if you don't know anyone, ask an esthetician to recommend clients to whom you might speak.

Getting first-hand information is just the initial step, however. Good results speak for themselves, but you your-self must also feel comfortable with a surgeon and have con-fidence in him or her. Interview at least three doctors and ask to see pictures of their work. Most surgeons require at least two consultations with a prospective client to ascertain compatibility and to make sure that she/he has realistic goals for the operation. It is not unusual to be charged a nominal fee (from $30 to $100) for this time. During these sessions, it's your job to ask questions. The more thoroughly informed you are, the less chance there will be for disap-pointment or surprise.

Before you consider surgery, you should know about nonsurgical alternatives that can improve your skin and appearance. Some of these treatments are new; others are thousands of years old. All of them are less expensive and less traumatic than plastic surgery. You may want to try one or more of them before going under the knife.

Home Improvement with Fruit Acids, Enzymes, and Oxygenation

If you have facial skin problems such as sun damage, discoloration, premature aging, deep expression lines, scar-ring, or loss of elasticity, you should first begin with my anti-aging skin-care program outlined in Chapter 13. The program includes the daily use of mild, natural products containing green papaya enzymes, betahydroxy acids such as willow bark, oxygenated moisturizers, and sunblocks. These breakthrough products, explained in Chapter 1, may be all that you need to correct skin problems. It may take regular use over a period of about 6 to 14 months to see opti-mum results, but if you use the appropriate products, you will begin to notice a difference in your skin in a matter of days. If you still feel you need more dramatic results, you may want to consult a cosmetic surgeon or dermatologist about a deep chemical peel or surgical alteration.

Chemical Peels: From Mild to Deep

There are various types of chemical peels, which work to rejuvenate the skin by peeling off old skin and shocking the development of new skin. The peeling process involves the application of chemicals to the skin, burning several layers of skin, and causing it to react as it would to a second-degree burn, producing collagen and new skin. The new layer of collagen that forms after a peel is thicker than the old layer. Thus, the peel tightens the skin and gives it a firmer stability. Depending on the strength of the chemicals used, the peel and the recovery process can be quite painful. There are three levels of peels: light, medium, and deep.

Light peels are usually done with a high concentration of alphahydroxy acid, such as glycolic or lactic acid. Light peels remove only the outermost skin layers, giving a fresh appearance to the face. They are effective on rough, dry skin, patchy pigmentation, and superficial acne scars. These mild peels will produce a tingling sensation, but they are not painful. Light peels can be done by estheticians as well as dermatologists. Some salons offer these peels in a series of five or six applications over a period of several weeks. The process may begin with nightly applications at home of an 8 to 10 percent glycolic acid cream and/or Retin-A, for two to four weeks. Then you begin the salon peel process, with a 30 to 50 percent glycolic acid concentration; that takes about an hour. There may be some redness and irritation, but no recovery time is required. The cost for a series of treatments (sometimes called "lunchtime peels") can range between $250 and $500. In my opinion, the same results can be had by using an AHA and papaya enzyme peel at home, daily, for several months.

Medium-strength peels are used for sun damage, fine lines and wrinkles, age spots, and light surface scarring. The peel involves a single application of a 35 percent concentration of trichloroacetic acid (TCA). Often a sedative is given to reduce the pain. *Deep peels* use higher concentrations of TCA or the chemical phenol and usually require anesthesia. Both of these types must be performed only by dermatologists or cosmetic surgeons. Both the deep and medium peels result in reddening, flaking, blistering, and scabbing over of the skin. These effects can last up to 10 days following the procedure. If applied too strongly or left on too long, the chemical peel may have other side effects. Uneven pigmentation and loss of pigmentation are common. Sometimes the face will be several shades lighter than the neck and chest. Also, the trauma of the peel can cause a herpetic breakout even in those not prone to herpes on the face. If such a reaction is not treated properly, scarring may result.

You can see, then, why it's so important to have medium and deep chemical peels done only by a skilled medical practitioner. The cost is between $1000 and $2000. Some cosmetic dermatologists are currently combining a light chemical peel with dermabrasion for a more controlled peel that can be concentrated or made deeper on certain areas.

The effects of medium and deep chemical peels last for one to five years, and the procedure may be repeated every two to three years. Most doctors agree that chemical peels are more effective than dermabrasion, though more painful. They also can be more dangerous because they destroy the pigment-bearing cells, melanocytes. With these cells gone, the skin's pigmentation is permanently lightened. For this reason, chemical peels are not appropriate for dark-skinned women. Any change in pigmentation makes skin extremely sensitive to ultraviolet rays; if exposed, brown spots or uneven pigmentation may develop. Skin that has been chemically peeled will never tan like unpeeled skin. However, brown spots that were removed by the peel will eventually return. Following a peel, a patient must avoid any exposure to the sun for three months. After that time, a sun-block with an SPF 15 or more must always be used.

Chemical peels can be incredibly beneficial to women with badly lined, degenerated skin. However, I would recommend consulting with a plastic/cosmetic surgeon or dermatologist rather than an esthetician, and I would not recommend this procedure for younger women who just want to get rid of a few superficial lines. Also, beware of at-home chemical peel products sold by mail order. If the formula is strong enough to work, it can also cause serious damage if used incorrectly. These are not products to fool around with, as they can permanently damage the skin.

Dermabrasion

Chemical peels are sometimes done in conjunction with dermabrasion, a method of removing several outer layers of skin by using electric brushes with fine steel heads. This process is sort of like "sanding" the skin: When the surface skin is removed, the shock makes the skin produce new collagen and new skin that is free of the wrinkles and scars. If you have deep acne scarring, other scars, or deep lines and wrinkles, you may be a candidate for dermabrasion, which must be performed by a qualified dermatologist or cosmetic surgeon.

If the entire face is being done, the process is carried out under general anesthesia. (Local anesthesia is usually used for small areas of the body.) The skin will look and feel badly burned for a few days and may be painful. Then it will start to "heal," with a crusty or scabby looking surface, for up to 2 weeks. Makeup may not be worn for 10 to 12 days following the operation, and complete healing may take up to 6 weeks. Because the new skin is pink and sensitive, you must keep your face out of the sun for at least 6 months afterward. The effects of dermabrasion can last up to 20 years, much longer than a chemical peel. Usually the procedure is done in the physician's office and takes about one to two hours. The cost ranges from $1000 to $2500.

Collagen Implantation

Collagen, the skin's primary structural substance, breaks down with age, leaving wrinkles and depressions in the skin. Now, collagen can be replaced by injecting it into the wrinkle crevice. Collagen injections are primarily used for deep wrinkles around the eyes (crow's feet) and the deep folds that extend from the nose to the mouth (nasal-labial fold). Natural collagen, extracted from the skin of cows, is injected directly into a wrinkle, depression, or scar, bringing the level of skin a bit higher than it was originally. Within 24 hours, the newly implanted collagen blends with that already present, and the wrinkles and lines are "plumped up" and less visible.

The problem with collagen injections is that the effects are temporary, and injections need to be repeated every 6 to 12 months. This can become an expensive habit, since the cost of one syringe of collagen is about $325 and the average initial treatment requires one to three injections, depending on the number and depth of the lines or scars being removed. How long the collagen lasts varies greatly, depending on a person's skin type, skin condition, and lifestyle. Usually, maintenance shots are required once or twice a year, and should be administered as soon as reversal begins, to avoid having to start all over again.

A product called Zyderm is most commonly used for the larger nose and mouth wrinkles, and Zyderm FL, an ultralightweight version, is used for fine lines around the eyes.

Before administering collagen, a physician must test you for possible allergic reaction. This is done by injecting a small amount of collagen just under the skin on the inside of the arm. The test area is watched closely for the next month, and changes are reported to the doctor. *Under no circum-*

stances should you allow anyone to administer collagen injections without this initial test. Unfortunately, there is still a 3 percent chance of allergic reaction in spite of negative test results. To be absolutely sure, you may ask your doctor to do an additional test injection on your face before proceeding with a total treatment. A new treatment under study is called autologen, which involves using a person's own collagen to prevent a possible allergic reaction.

Collagen injections are generally considered to be safe, effective, and inexpensive compared to cosmetic surgery. The only area in which I do not recommend using collagen is the eye area. The skin there is so fine that very often the collagen remains in visible lumps for as long as several months. If your doctor assures you that this will not happen, ask him or her to do one small test injection in the eye area; then wait two weeks to see your reaction.

One of the most popular uses of collagen is to plump up the lips. Initially made fashionable by pouty-lipped, high-fashion models, lip-plumping has become very popular among the general population. When collagen is used for this purpose, it only lasts from two to five months, making it a very expensive treatment to maintain. However, some recent controversy has arisen concerning the usage of collagen and a possible link to autoimmune disease. No conclusive evidence has yet been presented, but there are some who believe that such evidence is forthcoming. If you are considering collagen as an option, I advise checking out fat replacement as a safer alternative.

Fat Replacement

Fat replacement is a new technique that uses a person's own body fat to fill out lines, wrinkles, and scars. It can also be used for buttock, breast, cheek and chin implants. The fat is suctioned by syringe from an area where it is not needed, such as the buttocks or thighs. It is then injected into an area where it replaces lost collagen.

Fat replacement is thought to be safer than collagen or silicone because it utilizes a substance from the subject's own body, reducing the risk of infection or rejection. Initial studies showed that the fat was absorbed by the body more quickly than collagen, making it necessary to repeat the procedure as much as 10 times for the desired results to last. More recent statistics indicate long-lasting results after 3 treatments. Some doctors now believe fat transplantation can be permanent and have begun using fat to augment breasts and buttocks. One of the most popular places to use this particular type of treatment is on the hands, replacing the lost fatty tissue that makes hands appear old.

Pigmentation Correction

The most common pigmentation complaint that both men and women usually have concerns "age spots," sometimes called "liver spots." They are dark brown spots that appear on the face, the V of the neck, and the backs of hands. Their official name is *senile lentigines*, and although they are associated with age, they are not a result of it. Instead, they develop from exposure to the ultraviolet rays of the sun. By the time the brown spots appear, the skin has already been irreversibly damaged. To prevent further irritation, sunbathing and extreme exposure to sunlight should be avoided, and a sunblock should be used when exposure is unavoidable. Lesions of this type should be examined by a physician if they change in any way—become larger, thicker, or develop a crust, since this may indicate skin cancer.

Physicians have several techniques for removing such spots. *Electrocautery* uses a fine platinum needle with an electric current running through it to burn the spot off. Very little, if any, pain is involved, and the area will heal completely within seven days. This can be a safe, effective treatment for small lentigines.

Bleach creams are products containing 4 percent hydro-quinone. These are sometimes effective when used over a period of time (six weeks to three months), but a total sun-block must be used in conjunction with the creams, since they make the skin supersensitive to ultraviolet light. Although commercial bleach creams are sold over-the-counter, they are not as strong or effective as ones prescribed by a doctor. I do not recommend bleach creams of any kind, because the brown spots usually reappear after even the most minimal sun exposure.

Cryosurgery, performed in a doctor's office, may be the safest treatment to date. Liquid nitrogen is applied directly to the spots to "freeze" them. Within 3 days, a small scab forms. When it falls off, in another few days, the spot comes off with it. There is minimal discomfort during treatment, and complete healing takes place within 10 to 14 days. This treatment is not recommended for those with very dark complexions as it may cause a temporary loss of pigmenta-tion that may last as long as several months.

When I turned 34 and noticed the first age spots on my own hands, I began investigating *natural alternatives* and found several that appear to have excellent results. Most of the spots are gone, and a few are smaller and lighter than they were; no new spots have appeared. Many nutritionists and herbalists also believe that it is possible to treat age spots by using several different natural methods. Like most natural treatments, these are not instant cures, but they don't require local anesthetics, cost hundreds of dollars, hurt, or possibly leave scars.

Among the best natural treatments are alpha and beta-hydroxy acids and enzyme products, which, over time, will help pigmentation problems. Another is the topical applica-tion of squalane, a nutrient-rich oil extracted from olives. Apply the squalane to the affected area twice daily; results should be visible within three months. Another natural treatment uses the topical application of aloe vera in con-junction with drinking it daily. To try this treatment, apply pure aloe vera juice or gel twice daily to the affected area, and drink two ounces of aloe vera juice in a large glass of water, twice daily. The antioxidant vitamins A and E are also believed to help fight age spots from the inside of the body by countering the effects of photoaging, aiding the production of collagen, and helping the cell growth processes of the skin. Follow the dosages recommended in Chapter 5 and remember to allow at least three months before expecting results. You may also want to apply these vitamins topically twice a day.

Regardless of which treatments you choose, it is imperative that a full-spectrum sunblock with an SPF of 15 or more be used at all times on any areas with pigmentation problems. To ensure absolute protection of your hands, wear gloves.

When dealing with damaged skin, I always recommend trying the most natural, least expensive, least invasive treatment first. In most cases, the nonsurgical approaches outlined here can revive the damaged skin, but there is always the option of surgery for more intractable problems. Remember that neither these treatments nor cosmetic surgery can make your skin healthy. You will still need to eat a sensible diet, exercise regularly, and minimize the stress in your life in order to make the most of any treatment, surgical or not.

8   Treatment Treats for a Fabulous Face and Body

With so many choices in skin and body care, we could easily spend a good portion of every day simply trying to take care of ourselves. New Age health practitioners, salons, and spas offer a dazzling array of treatments for the face and body, all aimed at helping you look and feel younger. Many of these treatments are quite expensive as well as time-consuming, and while all of them may make you feel good, some are more effective than others for promoting skin health and preventing aging. Of the many treatment treats offered these days, I can recommend a few that I believe are the most worthwhile.

Deep Face Cleansing with Professional Facials

One of the most important treatments to keep your face looking younger is a professional facial. Ideally, you should get one once every month or at least every two months. Professional facials give your skin a deep cleansing that opens clogged pores and rids you of blackheads, whiteheads, and pimples without damaging the skin. Estheticians also offer professional quality exfoliation (peeling) using AHAs or enzymes that exfoliate the skin more thoroughly than the at-home products available.

The analogy I like to make regarding the benefits of facials is this: You brush your teeth twice a day, but still have your teeth professionally cleaned once or twice a year, right? We all know that a dental hygienist is able to give a deeper cleaning than you can get at home. The same principle applies to facials. In addition, an esthetician examines your skin using a magnifying apparatus in order to detect any possible trouble spots on your skin. She or he can identify dry areas that may be the beginning of eczema or psoriasis, age spots or moles, as well as precancerous lesions or skin cancers. All of these conditions respond best to treatment when detected at an early stage.

There are a number of different types of facials, and estheticians (like masseurs) have different styles and products they use. The two most important aspects of getting a facial are knowing the quality of facial you want and finding the right esthetician/facialist.

First, do not go to someone who uses a "vacuum" machine. This useless contraption does nothing but suck up surface dirt and break capillaries. Another thing to avoid are whirling, electric facial brushes. If too much pressure is applied by these, you could be red for hours. If excess pressure is applied to pale, sensitive skin or if the brush itself is too hard, capillaries may be broken, resulting in permanent redness. These brushes also aggravate oily skin by "exciting" oil glands to produce more oil. Those with problem skin should never submit their faces to this rough treatment because it is too irritating. Most respectable estheticians would never use either such machine, although some use a supersoft version of the whirling brush to remove cleansers from the skin.

Another way of judging the quality of an esthetician is to check out the products he or she uses and sells. If they are high quality, meaning natural and mineral oil–free, at least you know the esthetician is on the right track. Many small salons prefer to use "private label" products. These are made in bulk by cosmetics manufacturers and then sold to the salons, who put their own labels on the jars. The profit margin on these products is enormous, and many salons sacrifice quality to make money. If a salon sells this type of product, ask to see the ingredients list. If it consists mostly of chemicals and mineral oil or petrolatum, find another salon. If they refuse to show you an ingredient list, find another salon. An esthetician is only as good as the products he or she uses.

One of the best overall guidelines for finding a well-trained facialist is to seek out one that has been trained in Russia. This is not as difficult as it may sound, since so many Russians have emigrated to this country. To get an esthetician's license in Russia, students must first complete four years of premed training. This actually certifies them as the equivalent of our pharmacists. Russian estheticians prescribe and formulate treatment products for a wide variety of skin problems, including many treated by dermatologists in this country. In Russia, most cosmetics are custom formulated and sold by estheticians rather than sold in the mass market.

As you investigate facialists, you should be aware that professional facials are available in various styles. Until recently, the most popular way of referring to a thorough facial was to call it a "European-style facial." This type of facial involves cleansing the face with a facial cleanser and massaging it with one of several products. The massage includes the neck, shoulders, and upper back as well as the face, making the treatment very relaxing. Following cleansing and massage, the face is steamed with a very fine mist, produced by a vaporizing machine, for about 10 to 15 minutes. An enzyme exfoliant is usually applied during steaming and removed directly afterward.

The esthetician then cleans out the pores by gently manipulating the skin to force clogs out of blemishes. This is done by using damp Q-tips, or hands wrapped in cotton cloth. Many people mistake this procedure for "squeezing," because that's what it feels like. When it's done properly, however, the well-trained practitioner will clean out black-heads, whiteheads, and pimples without damaging skin. This is the only part of the process that may be painful or uncomfortable, depending on the depth and number of blemishes to be removed. If a deep blemish is opened and removed, the skin may be red and swollen for a few hours or more, following treatment.

Once the pores are clean, a mask is applied. This part of the procedure varies enormously from one salon to another, depending on the product lines used and skin type being treated. Masks may include the following:

◆ concentrates in the form of ampoules that contain a wide variety of botanical extracts, protein derivatives, vitamins, or lipids that are applied before, during, or after the mask

◆ strips of cloth that have been soaked in a solution of these concentrates rather than applying the product itself directly to the skin

◆ a soft, plastic face covering with electric current running through it that is placed over the face to assist nutrients to enter the skin

◆ latex-based mixtures that heat up and are brushed on to form a rubberlike mask that is removed in one piece

◆ a clay mask applied with a brush and allowed to dry and harden, then removed in one piece.

The possibilities are endless and continually changing as companies develop new products and procedures. A good esthetician will use a variety of different masks according to the needs of the skin. On one occasion she or he may apply a rich, hydrating mask, while on another a toning and firming mask.

Another style of facial is the "aromatherapy facial," which incorporates essential oils into most or all of the products used during the procedure. An aromatherapy facial helps relieve tension and stress, soothe sore muscles, and either relax or elevate your mood simply by the inhalation of fragrant essential oils. A well-trained aromatherapist will custom blend essential oils for your specific skin type. Many aromatherapists also blend personal products for at-home use. Long popular in Europe, this type of facial is beginning to become quite popular in the United States. It is my personal favorite, because it is customized for each treatment and gives such great results.

Aromatherapy and Essential Oils

Although you may first experience aromatherapy through the facial process, there is a great deal more involved in this field of body treatment. Aromatherapy is the art and science of using aromatic oils extracted from plants to bring about physical and mental healing. It is only recently that this ancient practice has become widely known and accepted in this country. Many consider aromatherapy a New Age phenomenon, but it is really just a new name for the process of using botanicals to heal—a process that is the oldest form of medicine known.

Five thousand years ago, Egyptians used plant-derived resins and oils in cosmetics, medicinals, and incense, and for the purpose of embalming. At the same time, the civilizations of China and India were also practicing aromatherapy. The Indian form has come down to us through Ayurvedic medicine, which has been practiced for more than 3000 years. The Greek Theophrastus experimented with plant extracts and their effects on thinking, feeling, and health, and by the third century A.D., the Romans had developed and expanded the use of aromatics, making them an integral part of pleasure as well as health. Fragrant oils were commonly used in baths, perfumes, and massage. The ancient Arabs, Aztecs, and Native Americans all used aromatics for medicinal and cosmetic purposes. In Europe, herbs were used medicinally for centuries until modern medicine began to crowd them out of the picture as a mode of healing. Still, modern aromatherapy continued to develop in France in the 1920s and 1930s, and has recently gained new acceptance by medical practitioners as well as estheticians.

The extracts used in aromatherapy are *essential oils* distilled from plants. In fact, they are not really "oils" at all, but highly volatile liquids that evaporate very quickly when exposed to either heat or light. They are called essential oils because the volatile fluids are generally infused into a base of vegetable oil. Partly gaseous and partly lipids, they are able to penetrate the skin more thoroughly than other oils or than water-soluble substances.

In addition to their ability to penetrate, the reason essential oils are so effective is related to the function that they serve within the plants from which they are extracted. Essential oils are the plant's immune system. In the plant, the oils float outside the cellular walls until the plant is injured in some way or until it suffers from being too dry, too wet, too hot, or too cold. Under such circumstances, the essential oils penetrate the cell walls and balance or heal as much as possible. After the essential oils have done their job, they are expelled and return to their former position, to be called upon again when they are needed.

The process is similar when essential oils are used on human skin. In high concentrations (10 to 30 percent), they penetrate the skin to heal the source of a problem such as dryness or inflammation. They work over a period of days to heal the problem, but should not be used continually once the condition has cleared up. In such high concentrations, they should only be used on an "as needed" basis or to retreat the problem, should it recur.

Each essential oil may have a variety of uses. Lavender, for example, is a gentle sedative that can also help relieve stress and nervous tension as well as promote healing of the skin. Rosemary, a stimulant, also aids concentration and is used to treat muscular aches and pains.

A number of essential oils are commonly used in natural skin care, and all of them work as antiseptics to help control bacteria:

◆ *For acne and oil control:* bergamot, cajeput, camphor, cedarwood, cypress, juniper, lavender, lemon, lemon grass, palmarosa, sandalwood, tea tree, thyme;

◆ *For broken capillaries:* camomile, camphor, cypress, rose;

◆ *For cellulite:* cypress, fennel, grapefruit, juniper, rosemary, tangerine, vetiver;

◆ *For dry, aging skin:* basil, camomile, clary sage, geranium, jasmine, lavender, lemon, neroli, palmarosa, patchouli, rose, rosemary, rosewood, sage lavandifolia;

◆ *For headaches:* camomile, coriander, jasmine, marjoram, rose, rosemary;

◆ *For humectant:* blue camomile, lavender, palmarosa, sandalwood, vetiver;

◆ *For pain relief:* birch, juniper, lemon grass, rosemary;

◆ *For rejuvenation:* jasmine;

◆ *For relaxation:* bergamot, lavender, melissa, neroli, pettigrain, sandalwood, ylang ylang;

◆ *For skin irritation and allergies:* spikenard, camomile.

Lymphatic Massage

In addition to the use of essential oils by estheticians for various facial and body therapies, there are other applications of aromatherapy. Medical aromatherapy involves giving essential oils by mouth as medicine as well as inhaling them through vaporization. Medical doctors in France are the most advanced practitioners in this field today, treating ailments from stomach ulcers to asthma. Holistic aromatherapy is a hands-on therapy treating various mind–body disorders and includes a detoxification process called lymphatic massage.

Lymphatic massage combines the healing properties of essential oils with those of massage. This type of aromatherapy massage involves the use of various combinations of essential oils, along with an appropriate massage technique, to help detoxify a person's body. It is therefore beneficial to the body in a number of ways. It stimulates circulation of the blood and lymph, stimulates the immune system, and reduces tension and muscle pain. Obviously, it can be very helpful in breaking out of the cycle of stress. Some practitioners do a series of treatments over a period of time aimed specifically at reestablishing the proper function of the lymphatic system.

The lymphatic system carries toxins and waste products in a colorless fluid called lymph. It flows through the smallest blood vessels (capillaries) into larger ones, finally arriving in the lymph glands or nodes where it is purified. During that process, the glands also use lymph to produce antibodies, which the body uses to fight infection. Once cleansed, the lymph reenters the bloodstream to once again begin its journey picking up toxins. Unlike blood that is pumped through the body by the heart, lymph is not pumped but is moved as the body moves. Inactivity or a diet high in toxins can produce an oversaturation of lymphatic tissue, which results in blockage of the lymph glands. These trapped toxins may then become surrounded with fat as the body attempts to protect itself. Keeping the lymph flowing properly is one of the reasons why regular physical activity is so important to the maintenance of health and beauty.

It is best to receive lymphatic massage from trained professionals, because they have the knowledge and experience to orchestrate the right blend of essential oils and massage therapy. If you want to learn more about it yourself and practice with a partner, you can get some of the basics from the book *Scentual Touch*. Written by Judith Jackson, one of America's foremost aromatherapists, this book teaches massage technique as well as how to choose and formulate essential oils.

Rejuvenating the Face with Acupuncture

Facial rejuvenation using traditional Chinese acupuncture has been in use for more than a thousand years. The empresses of China were known for their flawless, lasting beauty, and one of their best-kept secrets was an ancient acupuncture face-lift treatment. Court physicians were sworn to keep this treatment secret to prevent the masses from reaping its benefits. Fortunately, this policy changed shortly after the turn of the century, and dissemination of acupuncture in the Western world has made this method available to us all.

An acupuncture "face-lift" works by stimulating muscle tone, helping to increase blood circulation, increasing the flow of oxygen to tissues, and speeding the elimination of toxins from cells. All of this combines to help the skin function at its optimal level, thus reducing the overall effects of aging.

According to the principles of Chinese medicine, a healthy body is a body that is in balance, meaning energy flows appropriately through the five systems, or meridians. If energy is too strong or too weak in any of the meridians, the imbalance will result in a problem or illness. An acupuncturist balances the body by working on the meridians, stimulating them or calming them as needed. To do this, she or he inserts very fine needles into points along the meridians. In an acupuncture face-lift, needles are inserted into the hands, face, legs, and back. Patients may report some mild, stinging discomfort but no pain. Depending on the condition of the skin, a treatment called "moxibustion" is often used in conjunction with the acupuncture needles. The moxi is a stick of compressed herbs that looks like fat incense. The end of the stick is lit, then allowed to go out, and the smoldering end is held close to the insertion point of an acupuncture needle, or at a meridian point near (but not touching) the skin. The smoke from the herbs penetrates the skin and acts as a tonic to boost circulation. The treatment lasts from 30 to 45 minutes and usually has a refreshing and energizing effect. The acupuncture face-lift is performed over a period of several months, beginning with bi-weekly treatments for six weeks, then followed by once-weekly treatments, until the desired effect is achieved. The cost for each session ranges from $35 to $70.

While I have not personally undergone an acupuncture face-lift, I have observed the results on several people. One, a close friend who was 42 years old at the time of treatment, had facial lines, dehydration, and loss of skin tone. After treatment, definite improvement could be seen. Her face appeared less tired looking and more youthful, lines were softened, and the skin around her eyes was tighter. The effects lasted for about six months; then her face began to show some of its original symptoms. If she had not been a heavy coffee drinker, I believe the treatment would have had a more lasting effect.

The only hesitation I have about recommending these types of treatments is that they require maintenance, which can get expensive over a period of two or more years. However, if your medical insurance covers acupuncture treatments, the cost would be taken care of. Another facial rejuvenation technique based on the principles of acupuncture is the *acupressure* face-lift, which is explained in Chapter 9.

Salon and Spa Body Treatments

There are a number of other face and body treatments offered by salons and spas. The idea is not to do them all on a regular basis, but rather to try them out to see which ones you enjoy the most and want to incorporate into your own anti-aging program. These treatments include body sloughing, salt scrubs, herbal and seaweed wraps, mud baths, enzyme baths, body masks, and hydrotherapy massage for exfoliation, detoxification, and relaxation.

Body Sloughing   This is almost exactly the same as the treatment you do at home to remove dead skin and stimulate circulation. The only difference is that the back of your body receives full treatment. The practitioner may use more pressure than you would use on yourself, and the full treatment takes about 20 minutes instead of 5. It's very much like getting a Swedish body massage, except the masseuse uses a sloughing cream and a brush or rope mitt instead of her hands. The sloughing is followed by a shower and the application of a soothing lotion. Your entire body feels alive and tingles, and your skin will glow!

Salt Scrubs   The body is moistened, then massaged with either coarse Kosher salt or Dead Sea salt. Although a salt scrub does a thorough job of removing dead skin and increasing circulation, this is not a treatment for everyone, because it can be painful. Equally good results may be gained from any of the other methods mentioned here, without the discomfort of a salt scrub.

Herbal and/or Seaweed Wraps   The main purpose of wraps, the most gentle type of body sloughing, is to moisturize and detoxify the skin. But the active ingredients also dissolve dead skin cells, making wraps excellent exfoliants. A warm seaweed extract is either brushed, or applied by hand, to the entire body; the body is then covered with a light plastic sheet or similar waterproof covering and wrapped in warm blankets or towels for 20 to 40 minutes. Herbal wraps are almost identical except strips of cloth or sheets that have been soaked in herbs are used to wrap the body. As you lie wrapped, surface toxins are drawn from the skin, nutrients enter, and dead cells are dissolved. Excess water is also drawn out of the pores, giving a "slimming" effect. It can even minimize the look of cellulite, creating a smoother appearance to the skin and taking inches off your body. However, these effects are temporary and the original size and appearance will usually return within 48 hours. Both herbal and seaweed wraps are often combined with some type of body brushing or massage, making them extremely relaxing.

Mud Baths   One of the oldest types of body treatment known, mud baths were used by the Egyptian, Aztec, and Mayan cultures. The mud is usually made from volcanic ash taken from various sources around the world. It is mixed with water, very often from a mineral pool or hot spring, to form a thick mud. The mud is mixed in large tubs and is thick enough so that the body rests on the surface, rather than sinking. When you take a mud bath, you lie down on the mud, your head resting on a bath pillow. An assistant then covers your body with handfuls of mud, leaving only your face uncovered. A cold cloth is usually placed on your forehead, and you are left for about 12 minutes. The mud is not uncomfortably hot, and the heat seems to penetrate very deeply into your body. For this reason, the treatment has had great popularity with arthritis sufferers. Like the seaweed, the active ingredients in the mud dissolve dead skin cells, making this an excellent body-sloughing treatment. A good, long rest is usually required after a mud bath, as it is quite enervating.

Enzyme Baths   Developed in Japan, this new treatment uses a large wooden bin filled with a blend of cedar fibers and plant enzymes imported from Japan. When heated, the enzymes stimulate circulation and metabolism and are also quite relaxing. Before the bath, you are given a special enzyme-powder drink that serves as a digestive aid. After the bath, the fiber is brushed off your body outside of the tub, and you shower before undergoing a blanket wrap for 20 minutes. The heat and chemistry of the enzyme bath produce an experience that is both relaxing and energizing.

Body Masks   Sometimes called "hot fangos," body masks use a mixture of either mud or seaweed and paraffin. The mud or seaweed is mixed into melted paraffin, then poured onto large metal pans that look like huge cookie sheets. The mixture solidifies as it cools, then the slabs are reheated to about 102°F. For a hot fango treatment, you lie face down on a massage table, and the assistant cuts a piece of fango large enough to cover the area of the body that you wish to treat— for example, the neck and shoulders. The fango is then placed on that area and gently pressed to help it conform to your body. The particular type of heat generated by this combination of ingredients is able to penetrate deeply to relieve tense, sore muscles. The effect is very relaxing.

Hydrotherapy Massage   Hydromassage is done in a large tub filled with water that is slightly warmer than body temperature. The newer tubs have dozens of Jacuzzi® jets built into their sides and bottom. During the first phase of a hydromassage, you lie comfortably in the tub for 5 to 10 minutes while the jets gently help your muscles relax. In the second phase, a masseuse uses water from an underwater hose to massage every inch of your body, beginning with your feet and moving up. The water pressure of the hose is adjusted to your comfort level and the overall effect is a deep-muscle massage without any pain. Treatment lasts from 20 to 30 minutes, varying from spa to spa. Although some people prefer the hand–body contact of traditional massage, to my mind, hydromassage is the most comfortable deep-muscle treatment I have ever had. I felt that the masseuse was able to work much deeper using the water than would have been comfortable for me had she used her hands.

Although hot tubs, Jacuzzis®, and whirlpool baths can be relaxing, they are not considered hydrotherapy because there is no practitioner or masseuse manipulating your body in any particular way.

9 Easy Rejuvenating Exercises for Eyes and Face

Although professional facials and salon treatments are important to your regimen, there are also a number of ways you can care for your face yourself. One of the most important is care of the eyes, which, more than any other part of the face, often show signs of aging. In addition to daily care, there are exercises that will rejuvenate the eyes and tighten and tone facial muscles to keep these areas looking younger longer.

The Eyes Have It

Thinking of eyes as the "mirrors of the soul" may be more than a flowery, romantic notion. Our eyes are the most expressive part of our face, instantly communicating the full range of our emotions, from joy to pain. They are the first thing you notice when you meet someone and the aspect of the face that is usually most remembered. It's a shame, then, that they are also the first area of your face to show signs of age. The skin around the eyes not only is the thinnest on the entire body, but the eye area also lacks sweat or oil glands that provide natural lubrication. The muscle surrounding the eye, the *obicularis oculi*, is circular and has no means of cross-support. If any part of it is weakened, the whole structure of the muscle is affected. A simple gesture such as rubbing the eyes stretches the muscle, causing sagging of the entire eye area.

When you consider the various expressions that involve the eyes—blinking, squinting, smiling, laughing, frowning, crying, squeezing shut, or opening wide—it's easy to see why this fine, unprotected skin wrinkles and lines so rapidly. Don't worry, I'm not going to tell you to stop making those expressions (except for squinting and frowning). It's the unnecessary gestures that put stress on the eye area that you can do without.

Another enemy of the eyes is gravity. You may not think that you can do anything to counter the effects of this particular foe, but you can. A few easy-to-follow rules will help fight the effects of expression, dryness, and gravity.

Essential Dos and Don'ts for Eye Care

1. *Don't weaken the skin around the eyes by stretching the supporting muscle.* Stop any habit you may have that involves rubbing or pulling the skin around the eyes. Learn to use your fingers in the opposite direction to the surrounding muscle to prevent it from stretching. Always begin any operation such as cleansing or moisturizing by placing the finger at the outer corner and moving it inward under the eye toward the nose, then continue the circle around over the eyelid, coming back to the starting position.

2. *Do use your middle finger instead of your index finger when applying cream, oil, or makeup to the eye area.* The index finger is too strong and can stretch the delicate skin. Practice using a touch so light that the skin barely moves.

3. *Do lubricate the eye area twice a day.* This is one of the most important ways to fight the signs of aging. An eye oil or cream should always be applied following cleansing. See Chapter 14 for information about eye oils, creams, and gels, as well as specific product recommendations.

4. *Do sleep on your back.* This utilizes gravity to help fight under-eye swelling and discourages the formation of unnecessary lines. If you sleep on your side, use one of the special hollow-center pillows designed to keep your face from being squished.

5. *Do wear dark glasses whenever you are outside.* Wearing sunglasses not only helps to protect the eyes from ultraviolet rays but also helps prevent you from squinting. Squinting is responsible for many of the expression lines around the eyes, on the nose, and between the brows. There is no excuse for not breaking this damaging and unattractive habit. If you squint because of faulty vision, have it corrected with eyeglasses or contact lenses.

6. *Don't use tissues around the eyes.* Tissues are made from wood and actually contain tiny splinters that can scratch delicate skin. Instead, use cotton pads or balls when wiping or cleaning around the eyes. To prevent cotton balls from "shedding" onto your skin, roll the ball around between the palms of your hands before using.

7. *Don't use waterproof mascara on a daily basis.* This type of product is designed to adhere, making it very difficult to remove. Layers of lacquer build up with daily use, causing lashes to break and fall out under the stress. I prefer to use a mascara without lacquer, because it is easily removed and doesn't harm lashes.

Getting Rid of Eye Puffiness and Bags

No matter how hard we try, there always seem to be those mornings that we wake up with puffy eyes or dark bags under our eyes. They might be attributed to not getting enough sleep, having a drink or two the night before, or high salt content in the previous night's dinner. Menstruation, birth-control pills, allergies, and sinus problems can all cause water retention that results in eye swelling. There are a couple of simple ways to treat eye puffiness if water retention is the cause.

The method that works best for me requires two tea bags. (Any kind of black tea will do.) Put the bags on a saucer and pour a small amount of boiling water over them. Let them steep for a few minutes, then gently squeeze out the excess water and flatten the bags to spread the tea evenly throughout. Lie down, spreading a towel under your head to catch any drips, and place one bag over each eye. Gently press the tea onto the skin, and rest that way for 10 to 15 minutes. Follow by cleansing your face as usual.

Another method that works well uses slices of cucumbers in place of the tea bags. Take a quarter-inch slice of cucumber, cut it in half, and place half on the upper lid, half on the lower. Lie down and rest for 10 to 15 minutes. Follow by cleansing your face as usual.

There are a number of products that can help tired and puffy eyes. Dr. Haushka Cosmetics makes an herbal concentrate called Eye Freshener that is designed to be diluted in water and applied on a cloth compress. It is available in natural food stores and facial salons and is very refreshing. Kelemata, an Italian cosmetics company, offers another good de-puffer called Maschere D'Erbe that is available in some major department stores. Lily of Colorado's Sea Therapy Mineral Eye Gel Mask is a convenient way to reduce eye area puffiness. It's available by mail order: 1-800-333-Lily.

I designed an enzyme-based eye cream that helps to soften lines while it improves the tautness and coloration of the delicate skin around the eyes. Because it penetrates completely, my Enzymatic Eye Cream may be used by all skin types.

Please bear in mind that these treatments are designed for the person who experiences *occasional* bags and puffiPness due to water retention. Permanent swelling under the eyes may indicate an accumulation of fat cells. This is a hereditary condition that sometimes may be improved with diet modification and eye exercise but usually requires surgery. People with this condition should not use heavy creams or oils around the eyes because those can make it worse.

Quick Pickups for Tired Eyes

When eyes burn or itch from tiredness or environmental pollution, the fastest relief may be found by using *artificial tears,* eye drops that duplicate the eyes' natural lubrication. Most drugstores carry one or two brands of this nonprescription eyewash, which is used like ordinary eyedrops. Ophthalmologists prefer this type of product to the ones designed to take away redness. In fact, some doctors believe that the very products designed to rid the eyes of redness, if used regularly, may actually cause redness.

Another treatment that soothes burning eyes involves making a cold compress with a washcloth and covering the eyes for five minutes. Rewet the cloth and repeat for another five minutes. Wrapping a little crushed ice inside the cloth is fine, but don't use ice directly on the skin because it can break capillaries. A ready-made eye compress called Aqua-Pac is available at most department stores. This is a gel-filled plastic mask, the shape of a Halloween mask, that is kept refrigerated until needed. Wrap it in a clean cloth before using.

Another fast way to relieve tiredness of the eyes is so simple it can be done anywhere and takes only about a minute and a half. Rub the palms of your hands together while counting to 30. Close your eyes and place your palms over the eyes, resting the heel of each hand on a cheekbone. Cup the hands rather than press them flat, and hold that position for one full minute. Keep the eyes closed after removing your hands, then slowly open and blink rapidly a few times.

Yoga Exercises for Eye Strength and Clarity of Vision

For centuries, yoga has taught a few simple exercises that strengthen the eyes. Some practitioners believe these exercises can also help correct weak or faulty vision. To get the best results, you should do the exercises twice a day for three weeks, then once a day until the desired result is achieved.

To begin yoga eye exercises, sit comfortably in a straight-back chair, feet flat on the floor with one hand resting on each thigh. Close your eyes and slowly take a deep breath through the nose. Hold the breath for a few seconds, then slowly exhale through the nose.

Step 1: With eyes closed, focus your gaze at the space between your eyebrows. Hold for two normal breaths. Open your eyes and blink a few times, then close and repeat the inward gaze.

Step 2: With head facing forward, slowly move your eyes as far to the right as possible and hold for 5 seconds, then return eyes front. Now move your eyes as far to the left as possible and hold for 5 seconds, then return your gaze forward. Repeat the right-to-left movements three times, then close your eyes for 10 seconds and rest.

Step 3: Keep your head facing forward and move your eyes up, as if trying to look at the ceiling. Hold for 5 seconds, bring them back to the starting position, then move your gaze down, as if trying to look at the floor. Repeat three times, then close and rest. Remember to keep your head perfectly still and your neck relaxed throughout these exercises.

Step 4: Slowly roll the eyes clockwise, in a complete circle. Repeat three full circles, then reverse direction and make three counterclockwise circles. Close your eyes and bring them to the forward position.

Step 5:   Rub the palms of your hands together vigorously for 15 seconds to generate heat, then place them over your closed eyes, with the heel of your hand resting on your cheekbone. Rest with eyes covered for 30 seconds.

Step 6:   Make an X with your eyes by moving them diagonally from the extreme upper right to the extreme lower left, and vice versa. Repeat three times, then rest with eyes closed for a few seconds.

Step 7:   Make the letter U by first looking up to the extreme right, then dropping the gaze down, then up to the extreme left. Repeat three times from right to left, rest for a few seconds, then repeat three times from left to right. Close your eyes, rub palms together, and cover the eyes for 30 seconds.

Facial Exercises for a Smooth, Taut Face

Just as exercises can help strengthen the eye muscles, facial exercises can help keep the face muscles toned and taut and keep the face looking smoother and younger. We may think of facial exercises as stretching the muscles when, instead, they are developing them. Talking, laughing, grimacing, and making any expressions that call facial muscles into play take care of some of the exercise facial muscles need. However, I believe that spot exercise of certain muscles that don't get used enough can make a difference in the way the face ages.

There are 15 different muscles in the face, but exercising any one of them affects all the others to some degree. Still, it helps to isolate some of these muscles, flexing and relaxing them to increase blood flow.

Before exercising the face, cleanse and moisturize it. Be careful not to frown and squint as you do the exercises. It may help to do the exercises in front of a mirror until you are quite sure of what you are doing. The following exercises are designed to strengthen muscles without causing undue stress to skin or underlying tissue.

Upper Lip

This exercise is designed to plump up the *levator labii superioris* muscle that holds up the upper lip. Since one of the first signs of facial aging is the loss of a full lip line, this exercise can be very helpful. I have found it to be effective when performed twice a day for several weeks. When results can be seen, you may want to cut down to once a day or every other day. Once you become comfortable with how to do the exercise, it can be done almost anywhere without using a mirror. It is not necessary to lubricate the lips or face while doing this exercise.

To begin, look in a mirror and open your mouth into a large O. Don't stretch your mouth open as wide as it will go; instead, open it comfortably wide. Relax the lips. Focusing on the center point of your upper lip, try to move it out and down to the count of 10, until it feels as if it is curling over your teeth. Hold that position for 10 seconds as you slowly inhale and exhale through the nose. Now *slowly* release the lip, to the count of 10, back to its original position. Relax the mouth, then open it and repeat the entire exercise two more times. This should always be done in sets of three.

Tightening the Neck

This exercise helps to firm and tone the neck by strengthening the *platysma* and *sternocleidomastoid* muscles. To begin, sit comfortably in a straight-back chair and slowly lean your head back to look up at the ceiling. Open your mouth; then, to the count of five, bring your lower jaw up until your upper teeth rest inside the lower ones. Hold that position while you inhale and exhale through your nose to the count of five. Then slowly release the lower jaw to the count of five, and bring your head back to the starting position. Repeat the entire exercise two more times. No lubrication is necessary for this exercise.

Double Chin

This is another exercise for strengthening the *platysma* muscle. To begin, sit comfortably and tilt your head back to look up at the ceiling. Then open your mouth just enough to stick out your tongue. Stretch the tongue out as far as it will go, then attempt to touch the tip to the end of your nose. Do this to the count of five, then release to the count of five. Close and relax your mouth for a few seconds, then repeat the exercise nine more times. This should be done twice a day (or more) for several weeks, or until progress is visible. At that point you may cut down to once a day. It's easy to do this almost anywhere, since it takes very little concentration and doesn't require use of a mirror or moisturizer.

Toning the Eyes

Many plastic surgeons recommend facial exercise to tone muscles before and after plastic surgery. This particular one strengthens the *obicularis oculi* muscle that surrounds the eye, thus helping to prevent or reduce sagging and puffiness. Because this exercise requires a facial expression similar to squinting, I recommend lubricating the outer corners of the eyes and cheekbones with a moisturizer or eye cream.

To begin, place the tips of your index and middle fingers between your eyebrows and hold them gently in place to prevent frowning. Keeping your face forward, lift your eyes toward the ceiling. Slowly, to the count of eight, lift your lower lids to meet the uppers. Hold the position while inhaling through the nose to the count of eight, then slowly release to the count of eight. Blink your eyes a few times, then repeat the entire exercise two more times. Be sure to blink eyes between each set. This may be done twice a day, morning and evening.

Facial Toner

This exercise is designed to strengthen the *temporalis* muscle, which stretches from the crown of the head down over the brow, around the sides of the head to the tops of the ears. It is the muscle most responsible for "holding up" the face. I call this particular exercise "mental face-lifting" because it uses the brain (imagination) rather than brawn (muscle power).

To begin, lie down, relax your body, close your eyes, and picture the *temporalis* muscle as it is in your own head. Imagine that it is slowly being pulled up and back, over your forehead and behind your ears. You will feel an actual tightening, which increases as you hold this mental picture. Allow the tension to remain for one or two minutes, then relax and open your eyes.

That's all there is to it. Two good times to do this exercise are in the morning, before getting out of bed, and at night before going to sleep.

Nasal-Labial Fold

This exercise is designed to strengthen the two sets of *zygomatic* muscles that stretch from the upper lip over the cheekbones past the eyes. When these muscles begin to slacken, a line from the nose to the mouth becomes visible.

To begin, place the thumb of your right hand up and under the corner of your upper lip and gently hold the skin by placing the tip of your index finger over the thumb. Gently holding fingers in place, raise the cheek up into a smile to the count of six. Release the smile to the count of six, and repeat two more times. Repeat the entire exercise on the left side of your face. I prefer working each side of the face separately to make sure that each is fully exercised.

Do-It-Yourself Acupressure for Toning and Healing

In Chapter 8, I discussed the use of acupuncture, the ancient Chinese form of medicine, to rejuvenate the face. As you may recall, acupuncture is based on balancing the body energy that flows through a system of meridians. Acupressure is acupuncture without the use of needles. It works by applying pressure to the meridians in order to stimulate the flow of blood, oxygen, and nutrients to supporting tissues and muscles. The result of this increased circulation is greater skin tone.

The Chinese philosophy regarding acupressure meridians explains that each outward point corresponds to an inward one. According to this system, there are eight major organs inside the body—brain, spine, large intestine, stomach and sinus, bladder, triple warmer (thyroid, pituitary, adrenal), small intestine, and gall bladder. Each meridian point on the face corresponds to an internal organ, as shown in Figure 3 on the next page. Thus, particular problems on different parts of the face—such as blackheads, pimples, or discolorations—may indicate imbalances or malfunctions in the corresponding organ. Very often, the organ may be balanced simply by using the acupressure technique. You'll know that balance has been achieved when the external condition clears up.

All you need to perform the acupressure face-lift are your fingertips. Use the tips of your middle fingers or thumbs, and press gently on each point for seven seconds with about four pounds of pressure, then release. (To determine what four pounds of pressure feels like, practice pushing down on a scale with your fingertips.) The nice thing

Number on Face	Breakout	Corresponding Organ
1	Poor diet	Stomach
2	Poor elimination of toxins, lack of fiber, lack of friendly flora	Large intestine (colon)
3 (blackheads)	Insufficient digestive enzymes	Thyroid, pituitary, adrenal
4 (blackheads)	Poor metabolism	Small intestine
5 (pimples)	Poor diet, high fat content	Gall bladder
6	Stress	Brain
7 (jawline and neck)	Poor elimination of toxins, lack of fiber, lack of friendly flora	Large intestine (colon)

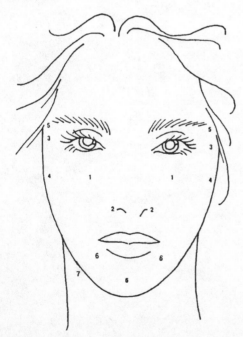

Figure 3
Breakouts and corresponding organs

about this treatment is that it can be done almost anywhere; try it in your car or while reading. It's very easy to incorporate into your daily life.

10   A Holistic Approach to Problem Skin

If you are blessed with clear skin that never breaks out, you can skip this chapter. But if, like most of us, you have encountered or continue to deal with problem skin of some kind, read on.

There are many different types of skin problems—excessive oil, blackheads, whiteheads, dryness and flaking, sensitivity, enlarged pores, rosacea (patches of redness), and adult acne—and not much awareness about the appropriate ways to treat them. There also seems to be more misinformation than useful information about proper treatments for these problems.

Oh No, Not Pimples Again!

In recent years, dermatologists have been seeing an increasing rate of adult acne in women. Most people believed that acne was behind them when they left their teens and early twenties, but now it is reappearing in their thirties and forties. While teenage acne breakouts usually occur on the forehead, nose, and cheeks, the telltale sign of adult acne is that it appears mostly on the lower cheeks, chin, neck, chest, and back (men most often get breakouts on the back). Also, adult blemishes and blackheads can be quite pronounced and often longer lasting.

Like adolescent acne, adult acne is the result of hormonal imbalances. Changes in hormones affect women particularly and at various predictable times in life—at the onset of puberty, during pregnancy and lactation, and at the onset of menopause. Generally, women are most likely to experience breakouts 8 to 10 days before their menstrual cycle begins. Add to this the other stresses of premenstrual syndrome, and you can have some real problems.

The hormone primarily responsible for adult acne is testosterone, a male hormone or androgen found in both men and women. The female hormone progesterone (which acts like testosterone) is found in some birth-control pills and can also be a contributing factor. Pimples occur when these hormones stimulate the skin's sebaceous (oil-secreting) glands and cause an irritation of the gland and follicle. As the follicular canal narrows, cells build up inside. Since oxygen can't reach the bottom of the follicle, bacteria breeds easily and pus forms, creating a blackhead, white-head, or pustule—different types of pimples.

Adult acne is the result of a number of factors that need to be treated holistically. Topical treatments alone may help symptoms, but unless the basic causes are identified and treated, the problems will recur. Other problems such as dry-ness and dehydration may occur as a result of many topical treatments because these products are designed to dry out pimples. The more effectively they do so, the more they dry out the healthy skin surrounding the pimple. In other words, treatment products applied to healthy skin create problems.

When dealing with skin problems, I prefer to address the causes rather than just the symptoms. There are, how-ever, some skin conditions resulting from psychological imbalance that need professional assistance. If you are suf-fering from severe skin conditions or experiencing symp-toms that do not respond to any at-home or salon treatment, I recommend that you see a qualified health-care practi-tioner or dermatologist.

If you have occasional breakouts, however, or if you have not yet tried a holistic approach, there is much that you can do yourself to keep your skin clear. Let's look at some of the major causes of skin problems and what can be done to solve them.

Stressed-Out Skin

As you may already know, stress is one of the major causes of skin breakouts and adult acne. It is also a factor in excessive oiliness. Stress-related breakouts of blackheads, whiteheads, and pustules usually occur around the jaw, chin, and mouth. According to traditional Chinese medicine, this area of the face also corresponds to the colon. Stress triggers a chemical reaction that creates a hormonal surge or imbalance. Most of us are aware when our skin is erupting as a result of intensified stress in our lives, and it's important to treat the source immediately. Otherwise, you may find yourself trapped in multiple successive breakouts from which you never get an opportunity to recover.

Treating stressed-out skin is similar to treating a stressed-out body, as I discussed in Chapter 6. Exercise is crucial to releasing tension and generating the beta-endorphins necessary to create a greater sense of well-being. Relaxation via deep breathing and/or meditation will calm you down and focus your energy.

Proper nutrition helps to combat stress by supplying the nutrients needed to maintain psychological as well as physical balance. Vitamin B complex, calcium, and magnesium are the nutrients that are most effective in relieving stress. Antioxidant vitamins, discussed in Chapter 5, are highly recommended for acne because they help to heal the skin and fight infection. Be sure to include at least 400 micrograms of chromium, 200 micrograms of selenium, and 30 milligrams of zinc. Give up caffeine and refined sugar, which cause extreme highs and lows in your metabolism and energy level. Caffeine is particularly bad for stress because it also depletes your body of the exact nutrients needed to fight stress!

But perhaps most important in dealing with stress-related skin problems is introspection. You need to stop and examine the reasons for the stress in your life, and then take action to alleviate those causes. If you can't rid yourself of the source of the stress, determine to counteract it as best you can. I know how easy it can be to put everything else before your own well-being, because I did it myself for years. After all, you can't neglect your family or quit your job. But in reality, you've got to make time to take care of yourself or eventually you won't be able to take care of anyone or anything else. Remember that your skin is a reflection of your well-being. If it is erupting, it is trying to tell you that something is wrong.

Diet's Role in Skin Problems

There are many theories about dietary connections to breakouts. Greasy foods, sugar, and chocolate are generally seen as the culprits. Even though the theories have not been proven, there is evidence that a diet high in fats and refined carbohydrates exacerbates skin problems. You should limit the amount of saturated fats and oils in your diet and avoid fried foods. Increase your intake of essential fatty acids (EFA) or gamma linoleic acids (GLA) as these are highly beneficial to the skin. Flax seed oil, evening primrose oil, borage oil, and linseed oil are all high in essential fatty acids. A reliable source tells me that the most beneficial and cheapest way to get EFAs is to grind up a tablespoon of whole flax seeds in a coffee grinder and ingest them with a smoothie, juice, or cereal daily. Follow the 10 Basic Rules for Anti-Aging Eating in Chapter 4, and you will probably see improvement in most skin problems.

In some people, iodine in the diet can be a cause of acne. Iodine quantities are particularly high in shellfish, salt-water fish, kelp, sea salt, and iodized salt. Red meat and dairy products are also high in iodine because of the iodized salt licks used for cattle and the beta-iodine solution used for sterilizing dairy equipment. To avoid iodine, substitute freshwater fish, tofu, beans, and free-range poultry as sources of protein in your diet. Use plain salt rather than sea salt, and use soya-based dairy substitutes in place of dairy products. Avoid products containing kelp, such as nutritional supplements, sushi, and food seasonings. Drink lots of pure water and herbal teas throughout the day to help flush out your system.

Poor Digestion and Elimination

Another major factor in skin breakouts has to do with what is called intestinal toxemia, or poor digestion and elimination. The resulting skin problems usually appear on the jawline, chin, around the nose, and at the temples.

Improving digestion is a matter of what you eat and what you don't eat. You will need to pay attention to your digestive process to determine what foods cause problems for you. When you experience indigestion, gas, or bloating after eating certain foods, this is a sign that your body is unable to digest them. Undigested food remains in the stomach or intestines and causes a buildup of toxic substances. Since the skin is the body's largest organ of elimination, it will attempt to get rid of toxins by causing breakouts. Try eliminating problem foods from your diet for a few weeks. If you still have problems with digestion, you may want to have a stool sample analyzed or take a battery of food allergy tests. See a doctor or a qualified practitioner for these tests.

The older we get, the more we become subject to food allergies. In fact, it is the foods we eat most often that we are likely to become allergic to. Wheat, milk, oranges, tomatoes, potatoes, and corn are the most common food allergens. Once these foods are eliminated from your diet, they can usually be reintroduced after a year or two without adverse reaction.

Another source of indigestion, gas, or bloating, may be caused by an inadequate supply of intestinal flora—the good bacteria that enable your intestines to break down foods. Red meat, alcohol, antibiotics, refined sugar, caffeine, drugs, artificial food additives, and other substances deplete the body's supply of friendly flora. To replenish your supply, take acidophilus with bifidus before meals. This combination of beneficial bacteria is designed to work on the lower bowel and liver and is recommended specifically for the treatment of acne. Regular acidophilus may also be taken after meals in place of an antacid to relieve indigestion.

Gently flushing the intestines is also important to rid them of toxins. As I mentioned in Chapter 4, there are many packaged "intestinal cleansers" on the market, but my favorite is the psyllium seed flush.

Aloe vera, described in detail in Chapter 5, is also an effective anti-acne treatment. Take it internally, three to four ounces in a large glass of water three times a day for 10 days, then decrease to two ounces twice a day for a month. Continue this dosage until the condition greatly improves, then cut down to one ounce twice a day until the condition is cleared. It is a good idea to continue drinking small amounts of aloe a few times a week to help prevent acne flare-ups.

Adding fiber such as whole grains, high-fiber cereals, Wasa bread, or rye crackers to your diet will also help your digestion. This natural bulk will help keep your digestive tract running smoothly. Fibercon and Crystal Star Chol-Lo Fiber Tone are over-the-counter fiber products that do not cause bloating like many drinkable fibers. For more on intestinal cleansing and detoxification, see Chapter 4.

Improper Skin Cleansing

If you have skin problems, take special care to cleanse your skin often and thoroughly to remove not just the daily dirt, but also excess oil, old skin cells, toxins, and bacteria. The longer these substances are left on the skin, the more trouble they cause. Bacteria thrive in a warm, moist (oily) environment, so cleansing the face twice a day is a must. Exfoliation should also be done daily but never with a granular (grainy) scrub, as these aggravate acne and excite oil glands to produce more oil.

It is very important to keep active problem skin as "calm" as possible, so a gentle exfoliant based on either natural betahydroxy acids such as cranberry, or green papaya enzymes is a perfect daily treatment. They digest only the old, dead skin cells without irritating the skin in any way. Also these vitamin-rich ingredients help to boost the production of new skin cells to repair redness, scarring, and old skin damage. Deep pore cleansing (another term for a facial) should also be done once or twice a week at home and once or twice a month by a professional esthetician.

You can give yourself a facial by steaming your face over a bowl of preboiled water with three bags of mint tea and a big slice of lemon peel. Place the bowl on your kitchen table, lean over it, and drape a bath towel over your head to make a steam tent. Stay there as long as the steam lasts (about eight minutes), then rinse the toxins from your face and apply a papaya enzyme peel. Leave on for 15 to 20 minutes. After removing the peel, apply a camphor-based mask to draw out more toxins and calm the skin.

Bad or Inappropriate Cosmetics

The kind of cosmetics you use on your face can be a big factor in skin problems, ranging from blackheads, clogged pores, and pimples to acne cosmetica—severe acne caused by cosmetic ingredients. Cosmetic acne is caused by comedogenic ingredients, meaning those substances that block skin pores and cause breakouts. Though it is not a true form of acne, since it is an externally caused condition, it is more likely to show up in people prone to acne—particularly if they are using the wrong products to treat their symptoms.

Although many products claim to be "noncomedogenic," you should read the ingredients list carefully because this term is grossly misused. If the product contains isopropyl palmitate or isopropyl myristate, don't use it. Other comedogenic ingredients to look for are mineral oil, petrolatum, cocoa butter, and coconut oils. If you're not sure about the ingredient listing, refer to the cosmetic ingredient dictionary at the end of this book. If you aren't sure about the ingredients, open the jar and try the product on the back of your hand. If it feels greasy, don't use it. A good rule of thumb is to avoid products containing oils of any kind. This means using a gel-based cleanser and moisturizer (if a moisturizer is really needed), water-based foundation makeup, and oil-free sun-care products.

When cleansing your face, remember not to use abrasive products of any kind. This includes buff puffs, loofahs, and wash cloths as well as grainy scrubs. Be mindful of using products that disturb the equilibrium or balance of the skin rather than maintaining it. In other words, use gentle, pH-balanced products rather than harsh ones. Avoid alcohol-based astringents that dry out the skin and fool the oil glands into producing more oil. Also beware of clay-based masks, because they draw all of the available moisture from the skin, causing surface dehydration.

When washing, massage your face with a cleanser and a little water for a full 60 seconds to help dislodge any oil and dirt from clogged pores. Always rinse your face with 30 splashes of warm water. Never subject skin to the extremes of hot and cold water. If you want to use an astringent after washing your face, saturate a cotton ball or pad and wipe it gently over the oily areas. Use the astringent once or twice during the day to prevent oil from building up. If your skin is combination, an astringent may be used sparingly on oily areas only. When spot-treating blemishes, use a camphor-based product or tea tree oil rather than products containing the extremely drying ingredient benzoyl peroxide.

Consulting a Doctor for Other Treatments

Once you have begun to address the root causes of problem skin, you can also examine other customized holistic treatments that may provide additional improvement in skin condition. I do not recommend antibiotics and topical chemical treatments unless the adjustments in your lifestyle and use of the skin-care program outlined above have failed to bring improvement. If you do need further help, you will probably want to consult a dermatologist about what is appropriate for you. Retin-A, antibiotics, hormone therapy, and accutane are part of the acne-fighting arsenal used by doctors. In some cases they are necessary to combat severe problems.

11 The Complex Truth About Cellulite

Cellulite (pronounced *sell-u-leet*) is a condition either experienced or dreaded by millions of women young and old, yet it is ignored in medical dictionaries and journals. Many doctors will tell you that it simply doesn't exist—that it is just another word for "fat." But those of us who have suffered from cellulite know otherwise. Even young, thin women with shapely legs can have what is known as "cottage cheese thighs" or have skin on the stomach, buttocks, knees, or upper arms that is bumpy or pocked in appearance—sometimes called "orange peel skin." Whatever the lumpy, rippled flesh is named, we certainly know it when we see it, and most of us are very confused as to what to do about it.

Why the mostly male medical world either has few facts or has little to say about cellulite is probably because it is a condition that affects only females. On the other hand, the beauty magazines and the cosmetics industry say they know plenty about cellulite, especially how to cure it in a matter of weeks or days, usually with a magic potion.

Myth and Misinformation

To give you an idea of the range of ignorance, myth, and misinformation about cellulite, here is a list of statements I have found over the years in medical journals, fashion magazines, health magazines, and books. Some statements are true and some are false. They will give you an idea of the extent of the controversy over cellulite:

- Cellulite is a unique physical problem with characteristics and treatments all its own.
- Cellulite is only a fancy name women have given to ordinary fat.
- Cellulite has nothing to do with being overweight.
- Being overweight is one of the initial reasons why cellulite forms.
- Cellulite is not affected by diet.
- A simple 14-day, lowfat, high-fiber diet will take it away completely.
- Cellulite goes away when you lose weight, but it is the last fat to disappear.
- To get rid of cellulite you have to reduce to three to four pounds less than your desired weight.
- Cellulite is not affected by exercise.
- Certain exercises such as leg lifts, tushy squeezes, hip rolls, aerobics, race walking, and swimming are sure cures.
- Cellulite is genetically programmed (inherited). If your mother has it, you'll have it.
- Cellulite is not affected by massage.
- Anti-cellulite massage is the fastest cure. Between 2 and 30 treatments are recommended, depending on the type.
- Cellulite will develop by the time a woman is 20 years old, rarely later.
- Cellulite develops when a woman ages, as a result of the natural slowdown in circulation.
- Cellulite is a result of poor circulation.
- Cellulite is a result of poor nutrition.
- Cellulite is a result of water retention.
- Cellulite is a result of hormonal imbalance.

◆ Cellulite is an overconcentration of fat cells due to a chemical imbalance in the skin cells.

◆ Cellulite is a different kind of fat.

◆ Cellulite is not fat.

◆ Cellulite is no different than any other body fat.

◆ Cellulite is trapped toxins.

◆ There is no such thing as cellulite.

◆ There is no cure for cellulite.

I have been following the cellulite controversy and doing my own research for more than fifteen years, and it seems as if every six months some new "authority" is interviewed regarding new findings or a new treatment. The authority usually proclaims that he or she has finally debunked the myths and found the solution to cellulite. These findings are diligently published in fashion and beauty magazines under such titles as "How to Banish Cellulite in Just 10 Days!" You'd think that by now there wouldn't be a single woman left in America with a cellulite problem!

The simple truth about cellulite is that it is a rather complex problem, one which does not lend itself to miracle cures or short-term treatments with magic creams. Cellulite can, however, be greatly improved and in some cases effectively eliminated by a combination of treatments: diet modification, detoxification, improving digestion, aerobic and spot exercise, and increasing circulation.

All of these topics have been addressed in this book, and the good news is that the recommendations I've given for preventing aging are the same as those for ridding yourself of cellulite. There is, however, some additional information that will be useful for treating cellulite. Let's look first at what cellulite is and what causes it, and then I'll set forth an easy-to-follow program to get rid of it and prevent it from coming back.

Cellulite: What It Is and Why Women Get It

The word cellulite, which is French, literally translated means "inflammation of the cell." Actually, cellulite has to do with the connective fibers that anchor the skin in most parts of the body. Located in the subcutaneous tissue along with the fat cells, they form a sort of honeycomb arrangement that holds the fat in place. When the connective fibers become thinner with age, the underlying pockets of fat cells begin to bulge through the walls of the fibers.

No one knows why some women get cellulite and some don't, but we do know that it only afflicts women. The reason women get cellulite and men don't has to do with the fact that women have more fat cells located in the subcutaneous tissue and also because the structure of the connective fibers is different. In women, the fibers are fewer and are vertical; in men, the connective fibers are more numerous and form more of a crisscross pattern. This stronger, crisscross design holds the fats cells down, whereas in women, the fat cells tend to bulge irregularly, causing the outer skin to look lumpy. Women's skin is also thinner than men's, and it gets thinner as we age. Also, our fat is distributed differently. Women tend to store fat in their thighs and hips. This fat storage is regulated by genes and hormones and is particularly resistant to slimming by exercise and diet.

Another factor in cellulite is the presence of toxins and the role of the lymphatic system in removing them. The rippling effect of cellulite is caused by fluid retention in adipose (fatty) tissue. Not only do the fluids cause swelling, but the toxic waste they carry becomes trapped in cells, causing the breakdown of collagen and elastin fibers. These swollen fat cells filled with trapped fluids and toxins create a blockage to circulation, another cause of the cellulite problem. When other cells are denied nutrients and oxygen because of poor or blocked circulation, they are unable to reproduce or function properly. This, in turn, contributes to the thinning of the connective tissue between cells and the further development of cellulite.

So while the actual direct cause of cellulite is the breakdown of the connective fibers, probably the biggest reason for this breakdown is poor blood circulation. When there is a loss of blood flow to an area—whether because of a poor diet (nutrient deficiency), clogged arteries, or a sedentary lifestyle—we have just the right environment for cellulite to develop. Once even a small amount of cellulite forms, it slows circulation even more.

In summary, the causes of cellulite may be broken down as follows:

1. genetic female fat cell and connective fiber structure
2. swelling of fat cells due to excess fat and fluids
3. breakdown of collagen and elastin connective fibers caused by trapped toxic waste, which results from poor circulation
4. thinning of cell walls and connective tissue due to the lack of nutrients (repair materials such as vitamins A, C, and E) and oxygen, which results from poor circulation.

It follows, then, that the "cure" for cellulite must address all of these factors.

My Own Experience with Cellulite Causes and Cures

I first noticed the beginning of my own cellulite condition when I was 36 years old. At that time, I had not been exercising regularly for several years and had gained some weight. I tried a couple of "cures"—first the Elancil Method, which gave no results, and then a series of massages that were supposed to "break up the hardened nodules of fat, water, and toxins." This was the most painful treatment I have ever had. Although it was called "cellulite massage," it contained none of the relaxing elements associated with other kinds of massage. In fact, I was black and blue and sore for the first three weeks of treatments. The pain alone should have made this the definitive cellulite treatment. However, the masseuse assured me that massage alone would not cure my problem: Proper nutrition and exercise were equally important. She told me that to banish the cellulite completely, I needed to lose two pounds more than my ideal weight and do an aerobic type of exercise for one hour, every other day.

I modified my diet to cut down on the amount of fat I ate. At the time, I was very fond of cheeseburgers for lunch, steak and fries for dinner, butter on everything, chunks of cheese for daily snacks, eggs and/or cheese for breakfast, and cream sauces galore. When I looked at my diet carefully, I was appalled at the amount of fat that it contained. I was also amazed, given that much fat, that I was only a few pounds overweight. Cutting out fat was an easy and effective way to cut calories and force my body to burn its stored fat. I was surprised at how quickly I lost my taste for butter, whipped cream, and cheese, all of which began to taste greasy to me.

I began an aerobics class and quickly became addicted to exercise, because I felt so good afterward. The first few weeks were killers, but when I began to see results, I wanted more. The combination of exercise, a lowfat diet, and the cellulite massage treatments did the trick. In about 10 weeks, I had lost my excess weight and the cellulite was gone. I continued eating right and exercising regularly for the next five years, and the cellulite stayed away.

I did not develop cellulite again until I was 41 and several aspects of my lifestyle changed drastically. First, I moved from San Francisco to Chicago, which automatically made me less active during the winter; I didn't walk as much and there were no hills to climb. Second, I stopped my usual aerobic exercise program. Third, I was writing two books, which caused me to spend up to 10 hours a day sitting at my computer; again, I gained weight. Fourth, I experienced the worst stress I have ever known for prolonged periods of time. You can see how these lifestyle changes related to the causes of cellulite:

Lack of exercise	=	Poor circulation
Sedentary habits	=	Poor circulation
Overweight	=	Fluid and fat retention
Stress	=	Toxic waste build-up

Two of these conditions—lack of exercise and over-weight—were part of my earlier cellulite problem. Sitting and stress added further to the problem, making the return of the cellulite worse than before. When I began my second program of ridding myself of cellulite, I was also writing *The Beautiful Body Book: A Lifetime Guide for Healthy, Younger-Looking Skin.* It was a perfect opportunity for me to test new products and treatments using myself as a "guinea pig."

Over the next few months, I tried a number of topical treatments that promised results within 10 to 20 days. These products were designed to be used at home and were marketed by some of the major cosmetics companies. I tried dry-brushing the skin, massaging it with a nubby plastic mitt, and applying exotic substances like ivy extract oil and seaweed gel. For months, I rubbed my thighs and but-tocks with various concoctions with names like Contouring Body Cream, Toning Body Oil, and Firming Body Cream. Although these products felt wonderful on my skin and were made with natural oils and botanical extracts, I saw no dif-ference in the appearance of my cellulite. Two other women testing the same products also reported no change in the appearance of their cellulite.

It seems a shame that these treatments are sold as mir-acle cures rather than what they actually are—adjuncts to a complete program of anti-cellulite treatment. Those of us who are truly concerned about our bodies would gladly use massage on cellulite areas every day for the rest of our lives if we knew it were an effective way to help prevent further formation. But we become discouraged by trying one method after another, expecting them to work overnight.

So what does a complete anti-cellulite treatment entail? As listed above, you will have to work on your cellulite problem on several fronts. The desire to get rid of cellulite can be a powerful incentive for you to undertake my anti-aging program. Not only will you eliminate those awful bulges, you will also find yourself healthier, happier, and looking great!

Anti-Cellulite Diet and Detoxification

Since we know that cellulite is caused in part by a combination of toxins, fat, and water retention, the nutritional guidelines are basically the same as those listed in 10 Basic Rules for Anti-Aging Eating in Chapter 4. Follow a diet that is low in fat, high in fiber, and full of foods that are as fresh as possible and contain no additives. If you are overweight and/or have pockets of cellulite, you will find that eating this type of diet will naturally cause you to lose weight without having to count calories. You'll also want to eliminate fried foods, fatty foods, red meat, sugar, salt, white flour, and artificial ingredients. Caffeine and nicotine are particularly bad for cellulite because they impede circulation and deplete your body of cell-building nutrients and oxygen. Alcohol should be kept to a bare minimum.

Follow the detoxification program described in Chapter 4 to cleanse the body of toxic wastes. This includes cleaning the intestinal track with a psyllium seed flush, replacing intestinal bacteria with acidophilus, and cleansing the blood with aloe vera. It's especially important to reduce water retention by cutting out salt and drinking plenty of water and herbal teas.

Keep in mind that you may experience some uncomfortable symptoms as a result of detoxification. You may also experience physical as well as psychological withdrawal from certain substances such as caffeine and sugar. When toxins that have been stored in your body begin to be released, they can cause nausea, headaches, stomachaches, backaches, exhaustion, pimples, and other uncomfortable symptoms. You may be irritable and even have trouble sleeping for a while. If any of these symptoms occur, just bear in mind that they are temporary and will disappear in a few days and that you'll feel a great deal better. Also, don't let yourself get stuck feeling deprived and denied. Remember that the detoxification process is temporary; you only have to be a "saint" for a week or two, then you can indulge your cravings for "imperfect foods" on an occasional basis.

The supplements you should be sure to include are the antioxidants discussed in Chapter 5 as well as a calcium–magnesium supplement for antistress and hormonal balance. You can also take a high dosage (500 milligrams) of niacin, which will help increase blood circulation. Be sure to take the kind that won't make you flush, or you could find the niacin very uncomfortable. Taking vitamin B_6 (100 to 200 milligrams daily) will help to regulate the water level in cells by maintaining the proper potassium–sodium levels in your body.

An Anti-Cellulite Exercise Program

Simply losing weight usually will not handle the problem of cellulite. To rid your body of cellulite, you must take up a program of regular exercise. Ideally, you should get some form of aerobic exercise for 20 minutes every day or at least five days a week. At a minimum you should exercise three days a week. Your program should include two elements—aerobic exercise and isometric or "spot" exercise. Whether you walk, swim, run, bicycle, or take a dance-type class, your aerobic exercise should be done at a moderate to low intensity in order to burn subcutaneous fat most efficiently. Conditioning the respiratory and circulatory systems also stimulates the lymphatic system to rid the body of toxins.

If you want the fastest possible results, the type of exercise that will have the greatest effect on cellulite is isometric exercise—the isolation and movement of one muscle at a time. This is easily accomplished with a program like Callanetics, which uses various isometric and stretching movements aimed at the problem areas of the body: stomach, "saddlebags," hips, thighs, and buttocks. See the Recommended Reading and Resources section for information about Callanetics books and tapes.

Another form of isometric exercise is strength training, which involves working out with weights and/or weight machines. If you do choose strength training, begin by working with a personal trainer who can put you on a program specifically designed for the problem areas you want to improve. Most gyms are well-equipped for women, and it's not difficult to learn to use the machines. Many gyms offer personal assistance at no extra charge.

It's always good to round out your exercise program with stretching exercises, including yoga positions that help keep your body toned and flexible.

Increasing Circulation

Another important aspect of an anti-cellulite program is increasing circulation with topical stimulation of the skin. This is where those ubiquitous anti-cellulite brushes and gadgets come in handy. But you don't have to use expensive products to get results. You can simply body-brush with a loofah, that rough-textured sponge or cloth for bath and shower. Scrubbing areas of cellulite with a loofah stimulates circulation, which brings oxygen and nutrients to that location. Be sure to let your loofah dry out after getting wet, or it will eventually mildew and fall apart. Dry-brushing the skin with a natural-bristle body or back brush also helps remove old surface skin and stimulates circulation; this should be done before bathing or showering. Ideally, you should dry-brush your cellulite areas twice a day using circular or sweeping motions toward your heart. If you have an Elancil gadget left over from a previous attempt, you can use it with body oil rather than the Elancil soap.

Salon Cellulite Treatments

You should make these do-it-yourself body brushings part of your daily care, but there are also several types of cellulite treatment offered by salons, including wraps, massages, and passive-stimulation machines. Most of these treatments are sold in a series of 10 or more because it is impossible to get immediate results.

The *salon wrap treatment* usually consists of:

1. exfoliation by brushing, loofah, cream, or seaweed;
2. wrapping in either an herbal mixture, seaweed, or special cream;
3. massage (optional);
4. application of a body lotion or cream; and
5. using a passive muscle machine at various times during treatment (optional).

Wraps alone are not an effective cellulite treatment; however, they work well when used in conjunction with diet modification (weight loss) and exercise. The effectiveness of a wrap treatment depends on the quality of the products used and the quality of the massage, but wraps alone don't seem to make a visible difference after the initial water loss has been replaced.

There are two types of *massage* specifically used for cellulite: lymphatic drainage and deep tissue; both are equally important. The lymphatic drainage helps to unblock lymph and create a healthy flow to release toxins and prevent further accumulation. Deep tissue massage helps to break up hard pockets of accumulated fat and toxins and increase circulation to blocked areas. The difference in the two is that lymphatic drainage is a gentle massage while deep tissue work can be painful and even cause bruising.

Passive-stimulation machines act on cellulite in several ways: They passively exercise muscles, which improves muscle tone and helps release toxins, and they help to break up fat deposits and increase circulation. There are many different makes of machines used in cellulite treatments, but all use an electric current with either electrode pads or probes. The electric current is supposed to increase circulation, break up the fat, and tone the muscles. The probe type is newer and less widely used, but seems to be more effective for increasing muscle tone. Keep in mind that machines using electrode probes are only as good as the technicians holding the probes. The machines may work for some people, but the treatments can be very expensive.

"Miracle" Fat-Reduction Cream?

Recently, two researchers announced a "miracle" cure for cellulite of the thighs, which has taken the cosmetic industry by storm. The product, which has been licensed to a company called The Right Solution, is a cream that contains 2 percent aminophylline, the active ingredient found in asthma medications. Scientists have known for some time that aminophylline, as well as a number of other substances, alters the fat cells, making it easier for them to shed their stored fat.

The preliminary study involved a group of 24 women who considered their thighs to be bulging and dimpled. They applied a topical aminophylline cream to one thigh and a placebo cream to the other for a period of six weeks. At the end of the test, the thighs treated with aminophylline were measurably thinner, some by more than half an inch in girth. This seems impressive, but the real question is whether continued use would reduce the thigh even further, as an inch or less may be barely noticeable.

There may be more questions about aminophylline still to be answered, however, it was recently banned for use in topical creams in Australia and is under investigation by the FDA.

One known drawback is that the cream does not permanently alter the fat cells, which means the effects will last only as long as the cream is used. Because the active ingredients do not enter the bloodstream, the manufacturers initially avoided screening by the FDA. Presently, the original formula for the product has been patented and only two companies are licensed to produce it. However, similar formulations have already flooded the market. I previously tested at least six with no consistent or positive results. Some seemed to work very slightly, but only for a short time, while others didn't work at all. However, I tested a product of this type that does not contain aminophylline but which produced extraordinary results. In a double-blind study conducted by a Florida physician, all eight participants lost a total of 34 inches from thighs, buttocks, waists, and abdomens. One woman even lost her double chin. The cream is called Sleek & Chic for women or Lean & Mean for men and is so effective that I have personally endorsed it.

Of course, if you are struggling with cellulite—just remember, no cream can affect all the complex causes of cellulite. And don't be embarrassed to ask for a refund if a product's claims fail to match its results.

12 Professional Makeup Techniques for Minimizing Aging

My approach to using makeup is simple: The older you get, the less you should use. As should be clear by now, the health of your skin is most important. If you take good care of your face and create balance and happiness in your life, that healthy glow will be the most beautiful "look" you can have. I'm not saying that you should go without any makeup at all. As we age, we sometimes need to enhance those aspects of the face that tend to "fade"—the lips, eyes, and the color in the cheeks. But rather than overdoing them, the idea is to restore them to their natural look. This doesn't take a great deal of time (who has time these days?). In fact, mature skin can be greatly enhanced by the simplest three-minute makeup, and if the proper products are used, they can help to protect the skin while making it look better.

When considering what sort of makeup you need, you may want to check out some fashion magazines to take a look at recent makeup trends. Don't be intimidated by makeup used specifically for photographic effect; instead, concentrate on makeup advertisements. Fortunately, as fashion magazines have begun to cater to the "mature" woman, makeup has taken a turn toward a natural and minimal look. Brightly colored eyeshadows and blushes are definitely a thing of the past. The current trend is to enhance rather than decorate. Too much makeup can emphasize lines and slack skin tone, giving you an artificial look and making you appear older.

It's easy to try out new makeup looks for free at your local department store. To introduce new products, major cosmetics companies regularly place makeup artists in stores to work individually with customers. Check with your local department store to see when they will be offering this service. It's a great way to find one or more new products that work well for you. You should be aware, however, that these representatives will want to sell you anything and everything. Don't feel obligated to buy, and resist the temptation to take home piles of products you don't need. You may find just one product that you like, or perhaps learn a technique you've never used before.

The following lists of basic and optional makeup products as well as some important tools for applying makeup should help you figure out your makeup regimen.

Basic Makeup Recommendations

Foundation

Eyeliner/eye pencil

Mascara

Blusher

Lip liner

Lipstick or lip gloss

Optional Makeup

Undereye concealer

Eyebrow pencil

Eye shadow

Face powder

Important Tools for Applying Makeup

Latex sponges for applying or smoothing foundation

Blusher brush

Pencil sharpener

Optional
Eye shadow brushes or sponge-tip applicators
Eyebrow brush
Large dome brush for applying powder
Retractable lip brush

Makeup Choices and Application

Did you know that the skin cells on the outer layer of your face are arranged in an overlapping pattern resembling shingles on a roof? Since the cells overlap in a downward direction, you should always apply foundation with downward strokes to get as smooth a finish as possible. The way you apply your makeup can be as important as the products you use. Here are some instructions for various types of products.

Foundation

When choosing a foundation, be sure to pick one that matches your skin as closely as possible. Don't rely on it to give you a rosy glow; that effect is best achieved with a blusher. A foundation is not meant to bring color to your face; its purpose is to even out your skin tone. An incorrect color will make your skin look artificial and will show a difference between face and neck. If finding an exact match to your skin tone is difficult, opt for the lighter shade as that will make your skin appear more even than the darker one, which can tend to make it look "muddy." Use a foundation that is lightweight, because the heavier it is, the more likely it is to settle into facial lines.

Apply your foundation by using the dot system. Using the tip of your middle finger or a Q-tip, dot foundation onto the chin, cheeks, and forehead. To spread foundation evenly, use either the tips of your fingers or a small latex sponge, and blend the foundation downward in the direction of your facial hair. This will flatten the hair and make it less apparent. The foundation should also be carefully blended to just below the jaw to avoid a visible "line."

If you use a latex sponge, be sure to wash it with soap and water and let it dry after every use so that it won't collect bacteria. (Bags of 25 to 50 triangular-shape makeup sponges are sold in most drugstores.)

Face Powder

Face powder helps set the foundation for a more lasting finish and gives the face a smooth "matte" look. It may also be used in place of foundation. Choose a noniridescent, talc-free matte powder, either loose or pressed. Apply with a large dome powder brush so that it goes on evenly and lightly. Too much powder can make the skin look crepey.

Eye Makeup

Eye makeup helps accentuate the eyes, enhance your natural eye color, and give the eyes a more "rested" look. The options for eye makeup include eye shadow, eyeliner, and mascara. All come in an enormous variety of colors. My personal recommendation regarding colors is to choose those that appear in your eyes. Eyeliner should match the darkest color that circles your pupil. Mascara should match your lashes, or be one shade darker if lashes are blonde. Eye shadow is an exception to the rule, as colors should be chosen to shade and highlight as well as enhance. The choice of eye shadow colors can depend on a variety of factors, including hair color and clothing as well as eye color.

You may want to consult a professional makeup artist if you aren't sure about what colors are right for you. She or he can also teach you the basics of makeup application as well as some of the newest options.

Eye Shadow

Eye shadow in powder form is usually much easier to apply and control than cream shadows. Powder blends well, making it easy to use two colors without looking obvious. Cream shadows stay in place better and don't collect in creases. To create a really soft, natural look with a cream shadow, gently smudge it with the tip of your finger immediately after application.

Always choose matte or translucent colors, never frosted or iridescent, as a shiny shadow will accentuate fine lines and give lids that crepey look. For the most natural effect, start with three colors from the same color family—light, medium, and dark tones. Apply the medium tone on the eye lid, the dark tone under the crease area, and the light tone on the brow bone. One of my favorite eye-shadow looks is to use the blush that you use on your cheeks. It is a quick method and very natural looking.

If your eyes are close set, apply the dark tone in the crease starting at the middle of the eye, working outward, and blend completely with an eye-shadow brush. Make sure that when you blend the dark color outward you sweep up toward the brow. If you blend downward, you will drag the eye down. If your eyes are wide set, apply the dark tone in the crease, starting at the inner corner of the eye, moving outward, but not going past the outer corner of the eye, and blend completely. This makes the eyes appear farther apart. If the eye shadow you are using is overly soft, apply it with a sponge-tip applicator so the powder doesn't flake off onto your face.

Eyeliner or Eye Pencil

The easiest form of eyeliner is a soft pencil that can be "smudged" and blended so that you don't have to draw an absolutely straight line. Liquid eyeliner will stay on better, but the line does not look as soft or natural. Some liquid eyeliners are now sold in something that looks like a felt tip pen, making them easy to apply.

Choose eyeliner colors that match the outer ring around your pupil. Stay away from "electric" colors, and opt for more neutral shades. Avoid jet black liner, which can make the eyes appear harsh looking. Instead, choose a soft black, brown-black, or grey-black. Also, stay away from iridescents, which can accentuate crepeyness. On the lower lid, keep colors light, as too much color under the eye can drag the eye down or draw attention to dark circles and bags. On the upper lid, apply liner close to the lashes, starting from the outward corner of the eye and moving inward. Soften the line by blending gently with a Q-tip. If using eye shadow, apply the liner after the shadow.

Where and how much eyeliner to use depends on the shape and "set" of your eyes. To find out whether your eyes are average set, wide set, or close set, measure the distance between them and measure the length of your eye. If the distance between is greater, your eyes are wide set; if it is less, they are close set; if it is the same, your eyes are average. For close-set eyes, the liner should start from the middle of the eye and move outward. For wide-set eyes, begin at the inner corner and move outward, stopping slightly before the outer corner. For average eyes, apply as you please.

Mascara

Mascara is used to thicken and darken the lashes. Black is the color most often used, but if you are fair-complected and your hair is light, you may want to use dark brown for a more natural look. My personal opinion is to only use black if your lashes are black. In the evening, you may want more than one coat, especially on the ends to lengthen them. But don't let lashes get "clumped" together—you can use a lash comb or brush to separate them.

I don't recommend using waterproof mascara on a daily basis, because it is difficult to remove and can damage your lashes, causing them to fall out. Use it only when you really need it.

If your lashes are very short or straight, curling them with an eyelash curler can make them appear more prominent. Start with clean lashes (no mascara), open the lash curler and then squeeze down very gently. Open gently as well, pulling slightly away from the eye. Make sure to keep the curler clean and to change the rubber pad periodically, because residue can adhere to lashes and pull them out.

Brow Makeup

The eyebrows are an often forgotten but very important aspect of makeup since they "frame" the eyes. To shape eyebrows, you may need to remove excess hair with tweezers or waxing. Unless you want to look like Madonna, you should retain the natural line of the brow and remove hairs only from under and between the brows. The lower part of the brow bone should be relatively free of hair, to give the eyes a more open look.

If you have ample eyebrow hair, you can spray a little hairspray on a brow brush then brush them up so that they stay in place throughout the day. There are now eyebrow tamers that come in wands like mascara; you brush a gel-like substance on the brows to hold them in place or to color them. If your eyebrows are very light in color, you can also define them with pencil or brush-on powder. If you do this, be sure to brush the brows to blend in the color. Another option is to have eyebrows dyed by an esthetician.

Blusher

Blusher is used to accentuate the cheekbones and bring color to the face. In choosing a blusher, it is very important to match the color tone to the natural blush of your skin. For example, if you have very fair, translucent skin with pink undertones, you would not choose a russet-toned blusher, which would work well for someone with golden skin. This does not mean you have to wear the same color of blush all the time—just stick to the same color family. The various families are: pinks, roses, plums, or mauves, which are blue-based; peaches, russets, bronzes, or browns, which are yellow-based; and reds, which can be either blue- or yellow-based. If you are undecided about which color category fits your skin, seek the advice of a professional color consultant or take advantage of the free color-matching service offered by Prescriptives, a makeup line found in department stores.

Blusher should be applied along the cheekbone. If it is applied too high, it will make the eyes look smaller; if too low, it can give the face a sagging appearance. Apply it after foundation.

With powder blusher, use a good blush brush to sweep the color along the cheekbone starting from the "apple" of the cheek out toward the ear. If the color is too intense, gently pick up the excess with a cotton ball or blend it thoroughly with your brush. I don't recommend using cream blushers, because almost all of them are poorly formulated, making them comedogenic.

Lip Liner

Lip liner is used to define the lips, correct uneven lips, and prevent lipstick from "bleeding." Lip liner should match lipstick as much as possible—no more than one shade darker. If you like using a lip gloss, choose a liner that is one shade darker than your lip color and blend on to your lips with your finger or a lip brush; then apply the gloss.

Lipstick

For the most natural look, your lipstick should be in the same color category as your blush. Some lipsticks last longer than others. In general, creamy ones will wear off sooner, but the long-lasting variety can be drying to your lips. To keep from getting lipstick on your teeth, use a trick some professional models use before a photo shoot: put your index finger in your mouth, close your lips around it and pull it out. This will remove any excess color from the inner part of your lips. Never use frosted lipstick, as it accentuates dryness and cracks in lips.

Makeup Techniques for Aging Faces

Several of the most common symptoms of an aging face can be easily corrected with the artful application of makeup—simple techniques you can do yourself that take only a minute or two.

Evening Out Skin Tone

Uneven skin tone is one of the easiest flaws to correct and makes a big difference in the way your face looks. The most common such problems are broken capillaries, darkness around the nostrils, a "valley" created by the nasallabial fold (nose-to-mouth line), and lines at the corners of the mouth. Let's look at these problems one at a time.

Broken capillaries are easily hidden by a good liquid foundation. However, if you have very large or prominent capillaries, you may need more than foundation. There are a couple of options to choose from. One is a green-tinted cream concentrate called a "color corrector." It's difficult to find one of these products that isn't mineral oil–based, so be sure to use it only when nothing else will cover sufficiently. To apply, tap or pat the base onto your broken capillary area, allow the base to set for a few minutes, then apply your regular foundation base as usual. The second option is to use an undereye concealer under your foundation base. Concealers contain more color pigment than foundations and thus provide more coverage. Apply in the same way as the color corrector.

Broken capillaries may be prevented or greatly improved by daily applications of the essential oil of cypress. You can make your own preparation by mixing one drop of cypress oil with one-half ounce of any light vegetable or seed oil, such as grapeseed oil. Apply this directly to the affected areas at bedtime. Or, you can use my Sea Tonic with Aloe Toner twice a day following cleansing; it contains the proper amount of cypress oil to treat broken capillaries. In either case, in about nine months, you will see a dramatic lessening of the redness caused by broken capillaries. Improvement will continue as you continue using products containing cypress. Just be sure not to increase the amount of cypress oil, as higher-than-recommended doses can be irritating to the skin.

Darkness around the nostrils is caused by two things: a group of broken capillaries concentrated in a small area, and/or the shadow of the nose. Either problem may be corrected by using concealer or base foundation one shade lighter than your natural color, over your usual base. When applying, don't try to rub or blend it with your fingers, or you may spread the lightness onto areas where it doesn't belong. Instead, use a Q-tip or fingertip, and tap gently to blend.

The *nasal-labial fold,* or nose-to-mouth line, is actually a shadow created by a "hill-and-valley" configuration. Applying a light concealer or foundation to the valley, over your usual base, will trick the eye into perceiving the area as a flat plane. Remember, dark makes things recede, while light brings them out. When you want to make a shadow disappear, always apply light. Again, use a Q-tip or fingertip and the tapping method to blend. The same principle applies to *lines at the corners of the mouth.* Patting on a light concealer knocks out the shadow made by the line.

Disguising Under-Eye Circles and Bags

This is a two-step process requiring light in one area and dark in another. The bags and puffiness are noticeable because they protrude, and applying a dark foundation will make them recede. It is easiest to use an eyeliner brush for application, since the area is small and you don't want to spread the "dark" away from where it is needed. Dark circles, on the other hand, are sunken, requiring "light" to bring them up. An undereye concealer one shade lighter than your foundation, applied very carefully with an eyeliner brush, will make these circles disappear. Always remember to press very gently in the eye area, since pulling the skin not only is damaging but will also spread products into areas where they don't belong.

A concealer should be moisturizing but not overly oily; a product that is too greasy will settle into the fine lines around the eyes. One of the best concealers is made by Prescriptives and is available in a variety of shades, which is unusual for this type of product. However, it does contain a small amount of mineral oil. If you have oily or problem skin or are prone to milia (tiny bumps) under the eyes, try the Origins product that is mineral oil–free. Both of these may also be used on eyelids to help eye shadow go on more evenly and stay in place without creasing. This can be especially useful for aging eyes, which tend to fold, causing makeup to gather in creases.

Bringing Out Bones

Using a highlighter to bring out your natural bone structure draws attention to the eyes and upper face and gives the face stronger definition. The highlighter is applied over foundation directly onto the cheekbones and is blended toward the temple. When light hits the bones, it is reflected, making them appear more prominent. A good highlighter should be slightly opaline white or translucent gold. Almost every cosmetics company makes one of these in either powder, cream, or liquid form. I prefer the creams or liquids because they can be blended into the skin, giving a natural look. For a more dramatic effect, try a gold or bronze powder.

Creating Strong, Youthful Liplines

Creating a good lipline only takes about 30 seconds longer than simply applying lipstick. This method will also help prevent lipstick from bleeding into the fine lines above the lips. (If you like using a lip fixative product, apply it first.)

Step 1:   When applying foundation base, include the edges of the lips.

Step 2:   Line the lips with a lip pencil either one shade darker than your lipstick or one that matches it, just slightly above your natural lipline.

Step 3:   Using a lip brush, apply lipstick sparingly inside the lines you've drawn, then blend the two together so that no harsh line is visible. If the liner and lipstick are the same color, you won't need to blend.

Minimizing Fine and Heavy Lines

Fine lines can appear anywhere on the face but are most common around the eyes and mouth. Pressed, talc-based powders, applied with flat powder puffs, emphasize these lines and can also be drying to your skin. If you like the porcelain look of powder, use a transparent one that is talc-free, such as my Natural Translucent Face Powder, applied lightly with a fluffy brush.

Heavy lines anywhere on the face may always be lessened by using "light." Think of a heavy line in terms of a hill and valley; if you lighten the valley, the shadow disappears. Any base or concealer that is a shade or two lighter than your natural skin tone may be used. Use an eyeliner brush to apply the light *in the line;* then, using the tip of a finger, gently press the color into your skin to blend.

Disguising the Double Chin

A double chin can be corrected by applying "dark" to make it recede. Blush or shader is the best product to use for this purpose; dark foundation is too heavy and tends to look muddy or dirty. To apply, look into a mirror and lift your head up. Using a large blush brush, apply the shading powder in an inverted triangle, starting with the point just above your Adam's apple, extending the sides out toward the corners of your jawbone.

Minimizing Drooping Eyelids and Crepey Eyelid Skin

These are problems that the wrong makeup can really emphasize. Here are some easy rules to follow that help to minimize this look:

1. Never use iridescent eye shadow; use pale translucent or matte shadows instead.

2. Moisturize the eyelids with a good nongreasy eye cream or moisturizer at least 10 minutes before applying makeup.

3. Use an eye primer/concealer before applying shadow.

4. Use a very pale shadow color on the bone just under the eyebrow, and extend the shadow out to the end of the brow.

5. Don't use eye pencil as shadow or liner, because drooping lids will cause it to smudge.

6. If your lids come down as far as your lashline, liquid shadows and eyeliners that are applied wet, then dry, are the only type of product that will stay on without smearing.

Products containing alphahydroxy acids make good treatments for the eyelids. *Just be careful not to get these in your eyes, because the acids can cause serious burns.*

Semipermanent Makeup

Makeup that is semipermanent—lasting one to five years—is one of the newest developments in the makeup field. Although the processes are somewhat expensive, they can be very good for women who are having increasing difficulty applying makeup or who don't want to take the time to do it daily. The technique is a type of tattooing that colors the skin semipermanently, lasting from one to five years.

Semipermanent Eyeliner and Eyebrows

This procedure originated in Japan, when a creative esthetician got the idea to tattoo "hairs" on a patient who had lost her eyebrows. It turned out to be a viable solution to this problem and is even recommended for women who have very light eyebrow hairs who would simply like to make them more pronounced. Later, the treatment was expanded to replace lost eyelashes.

A local anesthetic is usually used during the application, although some people do it without anesthetic. The treatment may be performed by doctors as well as estheticians, but this varies from state to state. In most cases, I believe that estheticians are better suited to do it properly because they have been trained as makeup artists and know what will be esthetically pleasing on different clients. I recall hearing about a mishap by one doctor who misunderstood what his client meant by "eyeliner" and tattooed a line, a la Cleopatra, that extended almost half an inch beyond her eye. This type of cosmetic enhancement is something you will have to live with for many years so be sure to choose your practitioner very carefully. Ask to view before and after photos of their work and have them draw the lines to be tattooed on you with lip liner or brow pencil before they begin the procedure. Choose a look that you are comfortable with rather than one they may find attractive.

Semipermanent eyeliner appears to be safe in all aspects. The dyes used are titanium dioxides and iron oxides and thus far show no sign of allergic reaction or toxicity. The only negatives may be that styles change, away from the eyeliner look, or that age causes the lower skin to stretch and droop below the lashline. In any case, only time will tell. The photos I saw looked just like women wearing different shades of eyeliner. If you are considering this procedure, ask to see some "before" and "after" pictures to get an idea of how this really looks; it is not a "natural" look, and it may not be right for you. It can also be used to fill in eyebrow gaps that may have resulted from scars, tweezing, or natural hair loss. Healing time is two to three days, during which time the area is usually swollen and scabbed over; then the scabs fall off.

Semipermanent eyeliner can last anywhere from one to five years, fading as time goes by. Touch-ups are recommended every one to two years to maintain the depth of color. The cost ranges from $700 to $2300.

Semipermanent Lip Lining and Lipstick

Semipermanent lip lining or lipstick is not simply an alternative to applying lipstick throughout the day. As we age, our lips tend to lose color and become thinner, and the lip lining technique can create a fuller line around the lips. You can also color the lips entirely so there is no visible outline when lipstick wears off. The shade used should match the darkest color present in the lips or be no more than one shade darker than that. This will have a natural appearance, and allows you to wear as little or as much lipstick as you like in any shade you choose. The cost of these processes ranges from $700 to $1200.

13

Easy Everyday Anti-Aging Skin-Care Program

One of the most important things you can do to keep your skin healthy and young-looking is to give it appropriate, diligent care. Now that you have general information about new skin-care products and treatments, this chapter provides a specific anti-aging program to follow on a daily, weekly, and monthly basis. This program will help you choose the products you need to establish your own skin-care routine. Chapter 14, "Product Information and Recommendations," will give you a thorough explanation of the products available and the ones that I think are best for various types of skin.

I don't know about you, but it seems to me that the older I get, the longer it takes to make myself presentable to the outside world. The days of jumping out of the shower, pulling on a pair of jeans and a T-shirt, and running out of the house with wet hair are definitely over for me. Yet none of us has the time these days to spend putting on our faces. The task at hand seems to be figuring out how to get the greatest results in the least amount of time. The program I present here represents what I think will produce the optimal results.

How to Determine Your Skin Type

Determining your skin type is the first step you need to take in beginning your skin-care program. You may already know that you have oily or dry skin, but taking the test below may give you additional information. Also, your skin may be changing. As we age, oily skin becomes less oily and dry skin becomes drier. All skin types become more susceptible to changes in environment and seasons. Each of the four basic skin types (oily, combination, normal, and dry) may also be considered "aging," sensitive, or problem skin— these are not skin "types" but rather conditions that may affect any type of skin. Daily cosmetics such as cleanser, toner, and moisturizer should be chosen according to your skin type, whereas treatment products should be chosen according to your skin's conditions. Traditionally, treatment products will vary and change more than the daily cosmetics you use, as your skin's condition will change more often than your skin type.

Following is a skin-type analysis involving a close examination of your face, three times in one day. Pick a day when you will not need to wear any makeup. In order to do the skin-type test, you'll need a nondrying gel cleanser, which you should choose from my list of recommended products. After you have chosen a cleanser, follow these directions:

1. Early in the day, wash your face and rinse well with 20 to 30 splashes of clean, comfortably warm water, then pat dry.

2. Don't put anything on your face following washing.

3. Wait two hours, then examine your face in a mirror, using good natural light. Now answer the questions in the checklists on the following pages.

4. Allow your face to remain makeup-free for the rest of the day.

5. At about 5:00 or 6:00 P.M., take another close look at your face in good light and answer the questions again. Notice if anything has changed.

6. Cleanse your face the way you did in the morning, rinse, and pat dry.

7. Don't put anything on your face before going to bed.

8. Immediately upon awakening in the morning, examine your face closely in good natural light. Answer the questions a third time.

First Examination—Two Hours After Washing

	Yes No (check one)			Nose Forehead Chin Cheeks (check as many as apply)			
1. Can you *see* any oil?	☐	☐	*Where?*	☐	☐	☐	☐
2. Can you *feel* any oil?	☐	☐	*Where?*	☐	☐	☐	☐
3. Can you *see* any dryness?	☐	☐	*Where?*	☐	☐	☐	☐
4. Can you *feel* any dryness?	☐	☐	*Where?*	☐	☐	☐	☐
5. Does the skin feel tight and look chalky?	☐	☐					
6. Does the skin feel tight and look smooth?	☐	☐					

Second Examination—Early Evening

	Yes No (check one)			Nose Forehead Chin Cheeks (check as many as apply)			
1. Can you *see* any oil?	☐	☐	*Where?*	☐	☐	☐	☐
2. Can you *feel* any oil?	☐	☐	*Where?*	☐	☐	☐	☐

	Yes No (check one)		Nose Forehead Chin Cheeks (check as many as apply)			

3. Can you *see* any dryness?   ☐ ☐ *Where?* ☐   ☐   ☐   ☐

4. Can you *feel* any dryness?   ☐ ☐ *Where?* ☐   ☐   ☐   ☐

5. Does the skin feel tight and look chalky?   ☐ ☐

6. Does the skin feel tight and look smooth?   ☐ ☐

Third Examination—The Next Morning

	Yes No (check one)		Nose Forehead Chin Cheeks (check as many as apply)			

1. Can you *see* any oil?   ☐ ☐ *Where?* ☐   ☐   ☐   ☐
2. Can you *feel* any oil?   ☐ ☐ *Where?* ☐   ☐   ☐   ☐

3. Can you *see* any dryness?   ☐ ☐ *Where?* ☐   ☐   ☐   ☐

4. Can you *feel* any dryness?   ☐ ☐ *Where?* ☐   ☐   ☐   ☐

5. Does the skin feel tight and look chalky?   ☐ ☐

6. Does the skin feel tight and look smooth?   ☐ ☐

You have *oily skin* if you answered

◆ *yes* to questions 1 and 2 and checked all four boxes.
◆ *no* to questions 3, 4, and 5.

You have *dry skin* if you answered

◆ *yes* to questions 3 and 4 and checked all four boxes.
◆ *yes* to question 5.
◆ *no* to questions 1, 2, and 6.

You have *combination skin to the oily side* if you consistently answered

◆ *yes* to question 1 and checked two or three out of four boxes.
◆ *yes* to question 2 and checked two or three out of four boxes.
◆ *no* to questions 3, 4, and 5.

You have *combination skin to the dry side* if you consistently answered

◆ *yes* to questions 3 and 4 and checked two out of four boxes.
◆ *yes* to question 5 one or more times.

You have *true combination skin* if you answered

◆ *yes* to questions 1 and 2 in the evening and/or upon awakening, and the boxes you checked changed.
◆ *yes* to questions 3, 4, and 6 one or two times.
◆ *no* to question 5.

You have *normal (or balanced) skin* if you answered

◆ *yes* to questions 1 and/or 2 upon awakening and checked one or two boxes.
◆ *yes* consistently to question 6.
◆ *no* to questions 3, 4, and 5.

Basic Rules for Oily Skin

Oily skin produces too much oil. To an extent, it can be balanced, internally as well as externally. Cut down on excessive oil and fat in the diet. Dairy products have an adverse effect on oily skin because of their high fat content. Switch to nonfat dairy products, or cut them out of your diet completely and substitute fat-free soy products and tofu (in place of eggs). Externally, discontinue use of all oil-based cosmetics, and

1. Stay away from rich, "super-fatted," oil-based soaps that contain coconut oil or cocoa butter, as these are too rich for your skin.

2. Never use oil-based "milky" cleansers, or any cleanser that is used without water.

3. Use an oil-free gel moisturizer in place of an oil-based one, as long as your skin is not dehydrated.

4. Use an aromatherapy treatment oil if the skin is dehydrated.

5. Use a mild, alcohol-free astringent during the day to help keep the skin oil-free.

6. Use a water-based foundation to help absorb oil during the day.

7. Use a nonabrasive exfoliant everyday to keep the pores unclogged.

8. Do not use "scrubs," because scrubbing activates the already overactive oil glands.

9. Don't use a loofah, buff-type scrubber, or wash-cloth; these collect bacteria and also activate oil glands.

10. Keep your hands off your face! (Bacteria are transmitted and thrive on oil.)

11. Choose a hairstyle that keeps hair off the face.

12. Don't use baby oil or oil-based cleansers to remove eye makeup (unless they are water-soluble).

Basic Rules for Combination Skin

Combination skin, as its name implies, is partially dry or normal and partially oily. Combination skin is usually oily in the "T zone," the area across the forehead, down the nose, and sometimes on the chin. It's usually normal on the cheeks.

1. If using products designed for oily skin, be sure to use them on oily areas *only*, and do the same with products for normal or dry areas.

2. Be aware, on a daily basis, of subtle changes in the degrees of oiliness and dryness. Most combination skin fluctuates, so your regimen won't be the same all the time.

3. Notice how changes in diet may affect the balance of your skin.

4. Use a cleanser that is gentle enough for the dry and normal areas but that clears the oil from the oily areas.

5. Use products designed to balance your skin.

Basic Rules for Dry Skin

Dry skin has a dull, chalky appearance and may actually flake off if gently scraped with a fingernail. It suffers from inadequate production of oil, dehydration (lack of water), or both. Beware of radical diets that eliminate all oils or all protein. Be aware of insufficient water intake and excessive amounts of alcohol, cigarettes, drugs, and caffeine. Externally, discontinue use of harsh soaps or cleansers and/or astringents. Avoid moisturizers containing mineral oil, and do not use abrasive exfoliating creams, masks, or scrubs.

1. Use an enzyme-based, nonabrasive exfoliant daily to help prevent the buildup of dead, dry cells.

2. Use a natural oil-based moisturizer that also contains humectants.

3. Never use clay-based masks, because they draw precious oils and moisture from the skin.

4. Use a specific blend of aromatherapy oils, such as Zia Aromatherapy Essential Oils for Dry Skin or for Hydration, to help boost oil production and help the skin hold moisture.

5. Use a liposome product under a moisturizer to provide deep, time-released moisturization.

6. Avoid any alcohol-based cosmetics.

Normal Skin

Normal skin has no areas of excessive oiliness or dryness. There may be light oiliness somewhere in the "T zone" (possibly by the end of the day and certainly during exercise), but it is never excessive. Normal skin is basically balanced throughout, but it is the skin type most susceptible to environmental and seasonal changes, becoming slightly dry in the winter and slightly oily in the summer. The most important thing to notice about this type of skin is that it can change slightly on a regular basis. Normal skin types may use either an oil-based or an oil-free cleanser, depending on how the skin feels that day. The same goes for a moisturizer. Usually, normal skin types use a lightweight, oil-based moisturizer, but in the summer, many switch to an oil-free gel. The general rule of thumb is to use balanced, gentle products on a daily basis and add treatment products as needed.

Skin-Care Rituals for the Face and Body: Daily, Weekly, Monthly

Daily Face Care

Morning

1. Exfoliation and/or cleansing
2. Liposomes and/or eye treatment
3. Toning
4. Moisturizing
5. Sun protection

Evening

1. Cleansing
2. Rejuvenating
3. Moisturizing

Morning Exfoliation

I believe that morning exfoliation is one of the most beneficial things you can do for aging skin and for repairing skin damage. I recommend that you use my 10 Minute Cranberry Miracle Mask every morning, followed by my 5 Minute Cranberry Neck cream to your neck. After five minutes, remove the neck cream with a wet wash cloth. Five minutes later rinse the mask from your face with warm water and cleanse as usual. My Cranberry Cleanser gives a second exfoliation.

Morning Cleansing

If you don't have time to use an exfoliant in the morning, use Cranberry Cleanser, leaving it on for one minute then rinsing it off. If you don't have time for either exfoliating product, begin your regimen with a thorough cleansing. Consult Chapter 14 to determine the best cleanser for your skin type. To get the most out of cleansing, always massage the face with an upward, circular motion for one full minute, using the soft pads of your fingertips. Then splash your face 20 to 30 times with comfortably warm water. (Remember, water that is too hot is dehydrating.)

Later in the day, if you take an aerobics class, run, or do something else that makes you perspire, it's important to cleanse your face afterward to remove sweat, oils, and toxins that have been released. If you're rushed or don't have your cleansing products with you, at least be sure to splash your face 20 times with warm water. It's not a good idea to let toxins, oil, and sweat remain on the skin as your body cools down—they will only cause trouble. The water also helps to rehydrate skin that has just lost a lot of moisture in the form of oils and water.

Enzymes and Eye Treatment

As I mentioned earlier, it is very important that something be used daily to treat the delicate eye area. Remember that the skin here is the thinnest on the body and lacks sufficient oil glands, making it the first place on the face to show signs of age. You cannot, however, use heavy, occlusive products around the eyes, as they will interfere with your makeup during the day and cause the eyes to swell at night. To moisturize the eye area, always use a water-soluble product that penetrates completely. Using the tip of your middle finger, apply the product from the outer corner underneath the eye toward the nose but not all the way to the inner corner as this can get into tear ducts and make the eyes burn. Also, be careful not to use any product on the eyelids that may run into the eyes. By applying products from the outer corner toward the inner, you will prevent stretching of the eye muscle, since this movement is in the opposite direction of the muscle itself. Oxygenated, enzymatic, and liposome products are excellent choices to use around the eyes because they penetrate so thoroughly and deeply.

Toning

A toner does several things: it tightens the skin, helps re-establish the skin's pH after cleansing, protects, and nourishes. Some toners also help fight bacteria and bring oxygen to the skin. Apply a toner with a cotton ball or pad or with your finger tips. If you use a spray-type toner, be sure to massage it into your skin with your fingertips. Toners are also refreshing and may be reapplied throughout the day by spraying over makeup. In fact, a spray toner will help "set" your foundation and make it last longer. When using this method, spray lightly from a distance and don't rub it in.

Moisturizing

Up until recently, in order for a moisturizer to work well it had to be applied on damp skin. The water (or toner) will help the moisturizer penetrate and "seal" moisture into the skin. If a moisturizer simply sits on the surface of the skin, it can only benefit the outermost layer of dead skin cells, and can also clog pores. This explains why mineral oil–based products don't work: they aren't water soluble and, thus, don't penetrate. However, the latest technology in skin care has produced "predigested oils" capable of penetrating dry skin completely. For this reason I use predigested oils in many of my new moisturizers.

Sun Protection

When the weather is sunny, wear a sunblock with an SPF 15 to 18 that offers both UVA and UVB protection. Use the block according to directions on neck, chest, and ears, as well as the face. If you have oily skin, choose an oil-free product. If you have normal or combination skin, the oil-free products will also work best for you. If your skin is dry, choose an oil-based product that will provide extra moisturization.

Because sunblocks vary greatly, it is important to follow the directions for their use. Chemical sunblocks are designed to be used before any exposure to the sun, which is why manufacturers instruct the user to apply them 15 to 30 minutes prior to sun exposure. Sunblocks that are not water resistant need to be reapplied frequently. All sunblocks protect you as soon as they are applied, but they should not be rubbed into the skin. In order to ensure proper protection they must be "laid on" evenly instead. If a sunblock is rubbed into the skin it loses about 50 percent of its SPF power. To work properly, both chemical and physical sunblocks must sit on the skin's surface. Many blocks are waterproof and won't be washed away by swimming or heavy perspiration. But waterproof blocks can cause clogged pores and should only be used when needed. If you use this type, you'll need to cleanse your face thoroughly after use. To protect yourself throughout the year from UVA rays (which penetrate through clouds and haze), you may want to use a foundation with sunblock on a daily basis. Once again, an SPF 15 to 18 is appropriate.

Evening Cleansing

A thorough cleansing at the end of the day or before bed removes makeup as well as dirt and toxins that may have accumulated during the day. It also prepares your face for any nighttime treatment. Use your cleanser, as you did in the morning, washing with an upward circular motion for one minute, then rinsing 20 to 30 times with warm water.

Rejuvenating

Nighttime is the perfect time to help your skin regenerate because this is the time when skin cells renew themselves most actively. But this is not the time for heavy, goopy creams. Several types of products are designed specifically for nighttime rejuvenation. Products containing natural alphyhydroxy or betahydroxy acids work well as do antioxidant creams and oxygenating moisturizers. Vitamin A, E, and C elixirs are good choices and may be used in combination with rejuvenating moisturizers for added effect.

Evening Moisturizing (Optional)

If you do not use a rejuvenating product, you should use your regular toner, eye treatment product, and moisturizer after cleansing.

Weekly Face Care

1. At-home facial
2. Masks
3. Essential oil treatments

At-Home Facial

Consider the at-home facial as a way of maintaining your skin between professional treatments. Not only is it good for the skin, helping to unblock pores and combat the effects of pollution and stress, it's a great way to relax as well. The facial has four basic steps. The products used in Steps 2 and 4 will vary according to the type of facial your skin needs at a particular time. The basic facial may be done once or twice weekly.

Step 1: Wash the Face.   Cleanse and pat dry as usual, but don't follow with toner, astringent, or moisturizer.

Step 2: Steam the Face.   The purpose of steaming is to soften the skin, open pores, and draw toxins to the surface. Plain water may be used, but for a more detoxifying facial, I find that adding a mixture of certain herbs makes a significant difference. The easiest way to get the right amount of the proper herbs is to buy one of two products—either Swiss Kriss, a laxative tea that combines 15 detoxifying herbs, or Crystal Star's Beautiful Skin Tea. Both are available in natural food stores as loose tea or in tablet or capsule form. The Crystal Star product also makes a wonderful facial rinse. Just strain the water used for steaming and use it to rinse your face afterward. You can also use mint tea as a steam booster; use two to three bags per treatment.

To steam your face, place two tablespoons or one tablet/capsule of herbs into a large bowl. Place the bowl on the kitchen table or any surface at which you can comfortably sit. Pour almost boiling water over the herbs. Sit at the table and drape a large bath towel over head, neck, shoulders, and bowl to make a steam tent. Don't get your face so close to the water or steam that it will burn. If the tent becomes too hot, lift the towel for a few seconds. This should be a relaxing experience, so it's important that you feel comfortable, breathe normally, and relax your face. Stay in the "steam tent" for about 5 to 8 minutes, or as long as the steam lasts. Rinse your face briefly with warm water or the strained liquid from the steam bowl.

Step 3: Exfoliation. This next step should immediately follow steaming. Now that your skin has been softened and your pores have been opened by the steam, you are ready to remove a layer of dead, dry cells, thus allowing deeper cleansing of pores. Use my 10 Minute Cranberry Miracle Mask and 5 Minute Neck Cream. Lie down and relax for 10 minutes. (It's perfectly all right to leave the neck cream on longer than 5 minutes.) Using a clean, wet face cloth, gently remove both masks, then rinse with clean warm water. Pat dry.

At this point your skin will feel silky smooth and soft; any whiteheads or blackheads that were brought to the surface by steaming should be gone, and circulation will have been greatly increased, causing a rosy, healthy glow.

Step 4: Apply the Mask. This is the final step of the facial, and the product you choose depends on your skin type and its needs. For oily, problem, and combination–oily skin types, the mask should calm the skin down by helping to tighten and close the pores. For dry and combination skin types, the mask should help to replenish moisture and oils, to help rehydrate the skin. Normal skin types should choose a mask according to the skin's particular needs of the moment. See below for information about masks, and consult Chapter 14 for specific product recommendations.

The mask is left on for 10 to 20 minutes according to its type, then gently removed by applying a wet washcloth directly over the face. Remove most of the excess using the washcloth and plenty of tepid water, then splash with tepid water 20 to 30 times and pat dry.

Step 5: Facial Finishing Spray.   This is an optional part of the facial, but one that I highly recommend. Use a simple solution made of essential oils mixed into water. You can purchase one of the facial spray products recommended in Chapter 14 or make your own by adding a few drops of essential oils to spring water or floral water and putting the mixture into a spray bottle. The oils you choose will depend on the type of skin you have and the effect you want to create. Remember to shake the mixture vigorously before applying and avoid spraying it into your eyes.

Facial Masks

Different types of masks are used for different results, and the type of mask you choose is determined by the effect you want. Traditionally, for oily and problem skin types, mud- or clay-based masks are recommended because they help to draw out toxins and to tighten pores. However, these masks are very drying to the skin because they also draw out moisture and natural oils. If a mud- or clay-based mask is allowed to dry completely on the skin (as most mask directions recommend), it will draw out so much of the skin's natural oils and moisture that the oil glands will begin to produce more oil to replace that which has been lost. This is exactly the opposite of what those with oily and problem skin need.

Unfortunately, mask manufacturers don't give proper directions on their packages; most tell users to apply a thin layer and let it dry for 20 to 30 minutes. This will totally dehydrate any type of skin! The proper application should be very thick—about one-eighth inch—and not be allowed to dry. If you want to use this type of mask, spray it with mineral water every few minutes, to keep it from drying.

Never leave a mud or clay mask on for more than 15 minutes. Those with combination skin should use clay only on oily areas, and normal skin types should use a clay mask for the sole purpose of pore detoxification (drawing out impurities). That should not be necessary more than once a month, at most. Clay- or mud-based masks should never be applied around the eyes, because they can cause stretching and severe dehydration of the delicate skin in that area.

Normal and dry skin types should use moisturizing masks, or those masks specifically recommended in this book for those types. Some moisturizing masks, especially those you make yourself, can be thin and runny. The best way to avoid making a mess with these is to lie down with your head on a towel-covered pillow to catch any drips.

Masks designed to tighten and "lift" the skin are an excellent choice to tighten pores or if your skin has begun to sag (lose its elasticity). When using a toning mask, keep your face relaxed and still while the mask is on. If this type of mask is drying to your skin, you may want to follow it with a moisturizing mask for 10 to 15 minutes.

You can also make your own masks at home using simple mixtures of fresh ingredients such as avocado, yogurt, oatmeal, cucumber, honey, fruits, and herbs. Vitamins E and A can be good additions to these masks, as can essential oils. Once you get the hang of proportions, you really can't go wrong. They are applied and removed the same way as a clay mask, though they tend to be thinner, and they remain on the face for 15 to 20 minutes. Think of natural masks as nourishing treatments, because the fresh ingredients are rich in protein and nutrients. I rely on them because good, clay-free commercial masks can be so hard to find. Here are two recipes for natural masks that I like a lot.

Avocado Mask (Normal to Dry Skin)

(Mix the ingredients together in a blender then add the essential oil.)

$\frac{1}{2}$ ripe avocado

$\frac{1}{4}$ cup plain yogurt

2-inch slice cucumber (peeled)

2 tablespoons honey

2 drops essential oil of lavender

Applesauce Mask (Oily, Combination, and Problem Skin)

(Mix ingredients together in a small bowl to make a paste.)

2 tablespoons fresh applesauce

2 tablespoons raw wheat germ

1 tablespoon oatmeal

1 teaspoon honey

2 drops essential oil of calendula

A wide variety of essential oils may be combined with mask ingredients to increase the efficacy of any mask. The following essential oils are excellent for balancing the skin and increasing hydration: palmarosa, geranium, lavender, camomile, rosewood, vetiver, and basil. To incorporate these essential oils into a facial mask, mix a total of 6 drops oil into 1 tablespoon of pure, cold-pressed oil (grapeseed, flaxseed, and evening primrose are best because of their high content of gamma linoleic acids), and add 1 tablespoon honey. Then mix this into 1 teaspoon of plain yogurt. This may be applied as is to your face and neck, avoiding the eyelids and leaving it on for 20 minutes, or it may be added to any homemade mask recipe.

Essential Oil Treatments

If your skin is extremely dry or dehydrated, a penetrating essential oil will do what a moisturizer never could. Essential oils, explained fully in Chapter 8, are used as a treatment for a period of 10 to 14 days. Their use should then be discontinued until they are needed again. Unfortunately, there are really no standard instructions that apply for continued use of essential oils after the initial usage period. "As needed" can vary enormously from one person to another. For some, it may mean using the essential oil treatment every two or three days, while others may need them only two or three times a month.

You can experiment with essential oils and create your own treatment products following recipes found in books on aromatherapy, try the pre-formulated products sold in health food stores and salons, or you can visit an aromatherapist and have a treatment product formulated specifically for your personal needs. Aromatherapy books are available in natural food stores as well as bookstores; see my list at the back of this book for those I recommend.

Monthly Face Care

Professional Facials

On a monthly or bimonthly basis, you should have professional facials, which are described in Chapter 8.

Daily Body Care

1. Bathing
2. Moisturizing
3. Exfoliating/dry-brushing
4. Sun care

From head to toe, the skin on the body varies through-out in degree of thickness and sensitivity. For this reason, different areas of the body require different types of care. Your daily body-care routine should include cleansing, moisturizing, exfoliating, and protecting from the sun when needed.

Bathing

The average American adult bathes once a day, or perhaps twice a day if he or she exercises. In their quest for cleanliness, most Americans bathe too much and use too much soap. If soap is used all over the body on a daily basis, the result will be dry skin.

Soap works by surrounding dirt, oil, and sweat so that they may be carried from the surface of the skin. But soap cannot discern between normal amounts of natural oils and other substances. Consequently, it also surrounds and washes away the body's natural surface oils. If a person with any type of skin other than oily washes with soap and water once or twice a day, the body may not have enough time to replenish its natural lubricants. This results in dry skin, itchiness, redness, sensitivity, a scaly appearance to the skin, dandruff, keratosis pylaris, and premature aging.

To avoid drying your skin out unnecessarily, use soap only where it is needed. Most people, washing in a morning shower, only need to use soap under the arms and between the legs. Only those with oily skin may need to use soap on the chest and back. Unless your body skin has actually become dirty or sweaty from working out, hard work, or nightsweats, soap is not necessary. Any gentle cleanser is preferable to soap, and a natural sponge or loofah used with plain water will do just as well.

Bathing Dos and Don'ts

Taking a long, hot bath is one of the easiest ways to relax at home; few things are as convenient and inexpensive.

Unfortunately, few things are as dehydrating. This need not be the case. There are several things you can do to make your bath beneficial to your skin as well as relaxing.

1. *Don't* make the bathwater very, very hot. The hotter the water, the more dehydrating it will be. Extremely hot water can also break capillaries, especially on the chest area, which is prone to this condition.

2. *Do* add bath oil to the water. This will help to make it less dehydrating. Instead of mineral oil–based ones, I prefer natural, vegetable bath oils because they contain valuable nutrients such as vitamins E and A. They also mix more readily with water. Mineral oil–based products float on the surface of the bathwater and are of no benefit to the skin.

3. *Don't* soak for more than 10 minutes in an oil bath unless it is of the aromatherapy type. Since there is no real value in a plain bath oil, the relaxation will come from being submerged in hot water. The addition of the oil is merely to make the soak less dehydrating to the skin.

4. *Do* use a bath pillow to support your neck and make relaxation more complete. These are sold in bath shops, pharmacies, and department stores. If you find it difficult to simply lie still in a tub, try reading. The bath pillow will make this easy to do.

5. *Don't* use bubble bath or foaming bath gels. These contain sudsing agents, such as sodium laurel (or laureth) sulfate, which dissolve the skin's natural oils. They may also leave a layer on the skin similar to that left by soap, if they are not rinsed off completely.

6. *Do* apply a body oil or lotion to damp skin directly following a bath. This helps to seal in moisture and prevent dryness. Choose a natural one that penetrates the skin easily, like Neutrogena Body Oil or Provenance Cranberry Lotion for the Body, or use one of the body lotions described below.

7. *Don't* use "bath beads." These are made of chemical salt compounds mixed with mineral oil and fragrance and have no value to the skin. They may also cause dryness if they are not thoroughly rinsed off. The exceptions to this rule are aromatherapy beads that contain pure essential oils in a vegetable carrier oil base. Be sure to read the label on any bath beads before purchasing.

Body Exfoliation

Whether you take a bath or a shower, it is important to exfoliate your entire body, below the neck, each time. Dry skin builds up on the body, just as it does on the face, changing its texture and appearance. Dryness, flakiness, "snake-skin" or "alligator skin," and a general dull, sallow look may all result from a lack of exfoliation. Regardless of the method used, always be very gentle on the chest area because the skin here is sensitive and prone to broken capillaries. There are several methods of exfoliation, although some are better than others.

Grainy or exfoliating soaps are bars of soap with some type of granule mixed into them. I do not recommend these because the soap makes them too drying. A *washcloth* is my least favorite type of exfoliant. It is not abrasive enough to be effective and can be a source of bacteria if used more than once. A *sponge* is my second least favorite type of exfoliant because it is usually not abrasive enough, can gather bacteria if not allowed to dry properly, and may fall apart too fast.

Because it is rougher than a sponge, a *loofah* makes an excellent exfoliator. Made of the inside skeleton of a dried gourd, a loofah looks like a strange type of sponge, and like a sponge, it expands and softens when it comes in contact with water. The open structure of the fibers allows air to pass through, which makes a loofah less likely to gather bacteria than a sponge or washcloth. A loofah should always be used wet, with circular, massaging motions. It is not necessary to use soap with a loofah. After each use, shake it out well and hang it up to dry; this helps to prevent mold and mildew from forming.

The ayate cloth is another excellent exfoliator. Made from fibers of the ayate cactus, the cloth has a big open weave that allows it to dry well and makes it easy to use.

Dry-brushing is another excellent method of full body exfoliation. In fact, it may be the most effective method available for at-home use because of the exceptional impact it has on circulation.

Dry-brushing, as the name implies, is done with a dry brush on dry skin. It must be done before bathing for approximately five minutes. Begin at the ankles, using short, sweeping motions toward the heart. Concentrate on areas of about 8 to 10 inches in length, moving up the body. Always brush in one direction only, toward the heart. Concentrate on the buttocks and upper thighs, especially if cellulite is present. You may want to ask someone to do your back for you.

When you first begin to use the dry brush, your skin may feel sensitive, but subsequent use will find it less and less sensitive. In fact, most people come to enjoy the feeling and find it to be quite invigorating. The increase in circulation also gives your skin a healthy glow.

The brush may be made of natural boar bristle, hemp, or synthetic fibers. Many of the dry brushes imported for sale in this country are too rough for the average American's skin. I tested several different types and brands and found the synthetic ones to be unbearably rough. Rope or hemp mitts are better than the synthetics but still quite rough. Boar-bristle brushes tend to be the softest and are still very effective. The old-fashioned, wooden-handled brushes found in pharmacies and bath and body shops are the best because the long handles make it easy to do your own back. When detached from the handle, the brush fits your hand comfortably, held on by its cloth handle.

Body Moisturizing

Apply a moisturizer of some kind after bathing, exfoliating, or dry-brushing. Chapter 14 gives complete information about the types of body oils and lotions available. Whatever you choose, always apply it all over your body after bathing.

Body Sun Care

In addition to wearing a sunblock on your face, you should also take care to protect the rest of your body from sun exposure. Please refer to Chapter 14 for my recommendations about sun-care products for the body. Most skin types can use less expensive, oil-based products on their bodies. However, if you have a tendency to break out on your chest or back, be sure to use the same oil-free product you use on your face for those areas. Mineral oil–based sunblocks can be used on all parts of the body except the face, neck, and chest; however there are many good products to choose from that do not contain mineral oil.

It's a good idea to use waterproof products only when they are needed, and to wash them off thoroughly as soon as you're out of the sun. Also, remember to reapply your sun protection product as often as the manufacturer recommends on the package.

Follow these basic sun-care rules:

1. During sunny weather, wear a sunblock SPF 15 to 18 that offers both UVA and UVB protection. Use the block on all exposed skin, including face, neck, ears, arms, and hands.

2. Use a waterproof sunblock when swimming, and reapply as directed.

3. Wear a hat of some kind, preferably with a brim to help protect your face.

4. Wear sunglasses with UVA and UVB protective lenses. The fact that these are now readily available in department stores and pharmacies illustrates the public's growing concern with sun protection.

5. Sit under a beach umbrella or in the shade to safely enjoy a beach or picnic.

6. Cover arms and legs with nonporous, light cotton clothing when walking, jogging, or bicycling in the sun for periods longer than a sunblock will protect you.

7. Walk on the shady side of the street and sit in the shady section of outdoor restaurants.

8. Protect your skin while driving—remember that UVA rays penetrate glass.

9. Use a lip block to protect lips, especially if you are prone to herpes.

Weekly and Monthly Body Care

Body Exfoliation

Beyond the daily care of the body skin, you should also exfoliate the body skin on a biweekly and monthly basis. Biweekly exfoliation, or sloughing as it is often called, is stronger than that which you do on a daily basis. It plays an important part in an effective body regimen because it helps to remove any residual buildup of dead skin and to increase circulation. Think of it as a more thorough type of exfoliation. Exfoliation is to your body what flossing is to your teeth.

Body exfoliation with a grainy, scrub-type product is easy to do while taking a shower. Stand in the shower and wet your body under the running water. Scoop a handful of the scrub mixture from the bowl and apply it directly to your body. Use both hands to gently massage small areas with circular motions. Work toward your heart, emphasizing the upward part of the motion. Remember to be extremely gentle on the chest area as this is prone to broken capillaries. Massage every inch of your body below the neck until all of the mixture is gone. This should take a total of three to five minutes. Step under the shower and rinse off completely with warm water. Follow with a cool rinse. Apply a body oil to your skin while it is damp, pat dry, then apply a body lotion. Your skin will be pink because of the increase in circulation, and should feel very smooth and soft.

Once in awhile, you may want to treat your body to a salon exfoliating treatment such as a salt scrub or body brushing. These are described in Chapter 8.

14 | Product Information and Recommendations

In the past decade, there has been an explosive proliferation of skin-care products for the face and body. The multi-million-dollar advertising campaigns that accompany these products make it sound like the fountain of youth has been discovered—again and again. Thus, it may seem almost impossible to know what products you really need, let alone which ones are right for you. If you were to believe the cosmetics companies, you might buy four different products just to get your face clean, and several more to tone, hydrate, moisturize, and ensure eternal youth. Applying all these products could take as much as half an hour, morning and night, not to mention the cost—often several hundred dollars! The saddest part, however, is that most likely you would not get the results you had hoped for.

This chapter is designed to help you navigate through the confusing world of cosmetics and skin-care products so that you can choose products that are well made and right for your particular needs. The information will also help you understand how some cosmetics ingredients can truly benefit the skin while others can actually be detrimental.

Reading the Labels

I encourage you to begin reading the labels of skin-care products, but until you become as familiar with cosmetic chemicals as you are with food ingredients, you'll find the labels difficult to interpret. That's why I am providing this comprehensive list of recommended products as well as a dictionary of cosmetic ingredients.

If you do feel inspired to get out your reading glasses and study a cosmetic-ingredient list, it's important to know that ingredients are listed in descending order according to their percentage in the product. Thus, the beneficial ingredients should be "primary" on the list. They will not, however, always be first on the list. In any product that is an emulsion (a creamy consistency moisturizer or lotion), the first ingredients will always be oil, water, and emulsifying agents. Then the beneficial ingredients should follow. Unfortunately, most cosmetics are not made this way. Because the beneficial ingredients are usually the most expensive, many mass-market cosmetics companies use only small amounts, while giving the impression that they use larger amounts. A perfect example would be a product called "Vitamin E Cream" that lists this ingredient as one of the last on its list. You may see aloe vera, camomile, azulene, and other precious ingredients used in the name of a product, when in fact they are present only in minute amounts.

At the end of the ingredient list should be the preservative system, two or more preservatives that work together to inhibit the formation of mold and bacteria. Preservatives are necessary in cosmetics to keep them safe. In fact, the more natural a cosmetic, the more it needs preservatives. Imagine mixing up a concoction of honey, yogurt, cucumber, kelp, and aloe vera juice, then dipping your fingers into it twice a day. You know you couldn't simply leave it on a shelf in your bathroom—it wouldn't stay fresh for more than a few hours.

To be effective, a good preservative system does not need to comprise more than 1 percent of a formula. Some preservatives can be irritating to the skin especially if more than 5 percent is used. Methyl-, propyl-, and butylparaben are, in my opinion, the most effective and benign preservatives, and are nonirritating if they account for less than 5 percent of a formulation. You can roughly estimate the percentage by their placement on a label. If they are the last ingredients listed, you can be fairly sure they will be well under 5 percent of the formulation. Natural preservatives such as essential oils, vitamin E, vitamin C, and grapefruit seed extract are effective but not effective enough to be used on their own in most formulations. The only exception to the preservative rule is the pure essential oil formulations that contain a variety of essential oils in a "carrier" or base oil. Almost all essential oils possess bactericide and fungicide properties and when used exclusively in a formulation will ensure proper preservation. Some enzyme products and AHA products are also stable without preservatives because of the nature of the ingredients.

Some cosmetic ingredients to avoid, especially if they are primary to a formulation, are mineral oil, petrolatum, propylene glycol, isopropyl myristate, triethanolamine (TEA), cocoa butter, coconut oil, and beeswax. Artificial fragrance and artificial color should be avoided even if used in small amounts, because they are not only sensitizing to many people but detrimental to our environment. When I began delving into and formulating cosmetics 20 years ago, most products contained mineral oil and/or petrolatum as a base. They were greasy and occlusive (remained on the surface of the skin), making them comedogenic (pore-clogging) as well as magnets for dirt. Tiny amounts of mineral oil in a cosmetic may not actually be that harmful, but so many cosmetics contain mineral oil—milky cleansers, moisturizers, anti-aging creams, eye creams, and foundations—that if you use a combination of these products daily, you are applying between four and six layers of mineral oil to your skin! I have found that when I take a woman off mineral oil–based products, her skin improves almost immediately.

In the past decade, the trend has been toward lighter products that penetrate the skin rather than simply sit on the surface. However, even some new, "natural" products contain occlusive ingredients such as coconut oil, palm oil, beeswax (only bad if a primary ingredient), and paraffin. Like mineral oil and petrolatum, these ingredients have large molecules, making them occlusive and potentially comedogenic.

Good natural oils used for cosmetic bases have small molecules, making them more closely resemble human sebum. This structure allows them to penetrate the skin and to impart their nutritional value of natural fatty acids and vitamins. Many natural oils also contain antioxidant nutrients such as vitamins A, E, and C, and gamma linoleic acids. Some examples are safflower, sunflower, almond, avocado, grapeseed, jojoba, evening primrose, flax seed, squalane, and borage oils.

Many products for the face now claim to be "cellular renewal" products aimed at speeding up the cellular renewal process. It is true that any product that remains on the face can assist in cellular renewal, depending on its ingredients—and on the amounts of those ingredients in a particular formulation. Cellular renewal ingredients include the antioxidant vitamins and minerals (vitamins E, A, C, beta-carotene, selenium, CoQ-10, germanium, ginkgo biloba, and squalane). Also look for retinyl palmitate, hyaluronic acid, NaPCA (sodium PCA), shea butter, linoleic acid (oils containing GLA), jojoba oil, mucopolysaccharides, triglycerides, wheat germ oil, gotu kola, avocado oil, aloe vera, and seaweed.

If you want to be sure to get your money's worth when shopping for cellular renewal products, the label should look something like this: Oil, water, lecithin, glyceryl stearate (or PEG-100 stearate), cetyl alcohol; these are the basic ingredients that comprise the emulsion. Then the beneficial ingredients such as aloe vera, vitamin E, squalane, and so forth, should follow. Almost all of the facial products recommended here are cellular renewal products.

Cruelty-Free Products

One of the things you may see on cosmetics labels these days is the term "cruelty-free." This certifies that the product has not been tested on laboratory animals. However, it may not guarantee that all of the *ingredients* in the product have not been tested on animals, since there are so many chemicals that have been tested that way over the past 40 years. Most cruelty-free products are natural, however, derived from benign sources.

You should know that the FDA does not require cosmetics to be tested on animals. During the past decade, new technologies have made it possible to use other forms of testing, like computer modeling and in vitro tests of cultured skin cells. Still, laboratory animal testing continues, although fewer animals are used. Many major companies in the cosmetics industry are no longer testing on animals, partly in response to consumer pressure and partly because animal testing is becoming obsolete.

There are a number of big companies who do test on animals, however, and if you want to be certain that the products you buy are cruelty-free, you should inquire about the maker's animal testing policies. You can contact the company's customer service line (the national directory for 800 numbers is 800-555-1212), or you can call PETA (People for the Ethical Treatment of Animals), a group that publishes a free, pocket-sized, cruelty-free shopping guide. Their number is 301-770-PETA.

"Green" Products

The term "green product" has come to represent any product that aims to be environmentally responsible in its production, packaging, and marketing. In the arena of skin care, "green" products would eliminate those that contain animal ingredients, test on animals, endanger the ozone, waste resources, or are packaged excessively. If you want to buy "green," you should look for products that use natural ingredients and take an ecological approach to packaging.

Cosmetic ingredients may be derived from animal, petrochemical, or plant sources, but I believe it is far more beneficial—both to the skin and to the environment—to derive them from plants. Using beef tallow to make glycerin, for example, requires far more water and resources than producing an equal amount of glycerin from coconut oil. With so many natural products on the market these days, you can easily avoid petrochemical derivatives such as mineral oil, petrolatum, and propyl alcohol, as well as artificial coloring and fragrance and unnecessary chemicals.

In order to conserve resources, we should also be aware of how a product is packaged. Glass bottles are generally more recyclable than plastic, but they are more expensive as well as being impractical for use in the bath or shower. And since glass containers are heavier, they use more resources in the shipping process. There are many different kinds of plastic, some of which are recyclable. In order to know if a container is recyclable, look for the recycle symbol, a triangular arrow with a number in the middle. But remember that recyclable products are useless if you don't make sure they make it to a recycling center.

You should also look for products that are packaged as simply as possible. Product boxes and product literature should use recycled paper and be printed with soy-based vegetable ink, rather than lead-based ink. In packing products for shipping, environmentally responsible companies use shredded paper, recycled shredded paper, or starch-based biodegradable "peanuts" rather than styrofoam peanuts. The styrofoam kind may be made with chlorofluorocarbons, or CFCs (the chemicals that are destroying our ozone), and they also take forever to degrade in our landfills.

Most important, if you see ways that companies could improve their packaging or their products, be sure to speak out. Federal law requires an address or 800 number on containers so that you can write or call.

About My Product Recommendations

The products I am recommending here have been researched and tested by humans to conform to certain standards of formulation and efficacy. The basic formulation standards are

- ◆ no mineral oil or petroleum-derived ingredients for the face
- ◆ no artificial fragrance or coloring
- ◆ no comedogenic ingredients
- ◆ the product is cruelty-free

If a product meets these standards, we then test it for efficacy. The testing program involves long-term use by a group of more than 30 people representing all ages and skin types. Products designed for specific skin conditions are tested by people with appropriate skin types and needs. The products recommended here are those that do not cause problems and, most important, do what they say they will do.

As a cosmetologist and cosmetics consumer advocate, my mission always has been to find the best possible products, and I'm happy to say that each year more and more products come close to this standard. As you will see from the product listings in this chapter, there are literally hundreds of good products available these days. I have included my own Provenance products, which are based on natural ingredients and geared toward skin rejuvenation. Obviously, I believe they are among the best on the market. In addition, some of my products are unique. I use cranberry concentrate in many products because it is a natural antioxidant and very high in vitamin C. My 5 Minute Cranberry Neck Cream contains an organic ginger concentrate to increase circulation and help rejuvenate the skin on the neck. My Oxygenated Enzymatic Eye Cream helps to regenerate the skin around the eyes in two ways: by bringing oxygen to increase moisture retention and helping to heal the outward signs of sun damage (discoloration, brown spots, loss of elasticity, uneven texture, and skin tone).

I have put all of the products into this one chapter to make it easy for you to refer to when shopping. Products are listed in the following categories:

Products for the Face

Problem Skin Products

Makeup Products

Products for the Body

Sun-Care Products (including both face and body)

These symbols denote where products may be purchased:

NFS = natural foods store

P   = pharmacy/drugstore

S   = salon

DS   = department store

BS   = beauty supply or cosmetic specialty store

MO = mail order

CR   = company representative

RX   = prescription

I   = Internet

Products for the Face

About Face Cleansers

There are different types of facial cleansers formulated for different skin types. Oil-based or creamy cleansers are appropriate for dry or normal skin, while oil-free cleansers work best for oily, combination, and problem skin.

Oil-Based Cleansers

There are two types of oil-based cleansers: those formulated with mineral oil that are massaged onto the skin and then tissued off, and natural oil cleansers that are water-soluble and are washed off. I do not recommend any mineral oil cleansers. The main purpose of this type of cleanser is to dissolve makeup. Many companies sell them accompanied by a "toner" or "freshening lotion" designed to be used after the cleanser. These are applied with cotton and actually remove the residue of cleanser, dirt, and mineral oil that has been left on the skin. A certain amount of the oil remains on the skin, however, and can cause clogged pores that result in blackheads, whiteheads, and skin bumps, and may also act as a magnet for dirt. In my opinion, this is an ineffective and potentially problematic method of cleansing.

I do, however, recommend good-quality, oil-based cleansers made with natural oils for people with dry or normal skin, especially those who like the feel of an emollient lotion-type cleanser.

Oil-Based Cleanser Recommendations

Annemarie Borlind LL Bi-Aktiv Cleansing Milk	NFS, MO (800-447-7024)
Botanics of California Chamomile Cleanser	NFS
Desert Essence Facial Cleanser	NFS
Dr. Hauschka Cleansing Cream	NFS
Earth Science A-D-E Creamy Cleansing Cream	NFS
Geremy Rose Santa Ana Cleanser	NFS

M.A.C. pH Balanced Cleanser	DS
Paul Penders Rosemary Elderflower Cleansing Milk	NFS
Provenance Cranberry Facial Cleanser	NFS, BS, I, MO (888-3ADVICE)
BorgheseTerme Di Montecatini Clarifying Cleansing Cream	DS
Zia Cosmetics Moisturizing Cleanser	NFS, MO (800-334-7546)

Oil-Free Cleansers

There are also two types of oil-free cleansers—foaming cleansers and cleansing gels. I generally do not recommend foaming cleansers as they contain detergents that serve as the foaming agent. The detergents commonly used—sodium lauryl sulfate, sodium laureth sulfate, and cocamide DEA—strip the skin of its natural oils, causing dehydration and fooling the oil glands into producing more oil. There are a few good foaming cleaners on the market that do not contain detergents, but I prefer to recommend cleansing gels that cleanse the skin just as effectively but use gentle ingredients such as aloe vera and citrus extracts. The gels will not strip the skin of oils and they have a low pH, which actually makes them good for all skin types.

Oil-Free Cleanser Recommendations

Foaming

Clarins Gentle Foaming Cleanser	DS
Earth Science Clarifying Facial Wash	NFS
Estee Lauder Thorough Cleansing Gel	DS
M.A.C. Foaming Cleanser	DS

Gel

Aqualin Cleanser	NFS
Cleanzyme	NFS, MO (800-800-0905)
Zia Cosmetics Absolutely Pure Aloe & Citrus Wash	NFS, MO (800-334-7546)
PrimeZyme Oxygenated Papaya Cleanser	NFS, BS, I, MO (888-3ADVICE)

About Exfoliating/Rejuvenating Products

In Chapter 1, I provided extensive information about the benefits of exfoliating and rejuvenating products such as AHAs—alphahydroxy acids or fruit acid products—and enzyme peel products. The following are my recommendations for products I believe really work to rejuvenate the skin without causing irritation. Remember that AHA products may cause breakouts. If this occurs, you can continue usage and get the breakout over with or you can switch to a betahydroxy product. If the breakouts persist while using an AHA product, definitely use the gentler BHA product.

Alphahydroxy Acid (Fruit Acid) Recommendations

Linda Sy Facial Lotion With Lactic Acid	MO (in California, call 800-232-DERM; outside California, call 800-422-DERM)
New Feeling	NFS
Origins Starting Over	DS
Paul Penders Herbal Citrus Exfoliant or Glycofruit	NFS
Provenance Willow Bark Beta Cream	NFS, BS, I, MO (888-3ADVICE)
Provenance Vitamin A Elixer	(see above)

Enzyme Exfoliant Recommendations

PrimeZyme Green Payaya Puree Mask	(see above)
Zia Cosmetics Fresh Papaya Enzyme Peel	NFS, MO (800-334-7546)
PrimeZyme Oxygenating Papaya Cleanser	NFS, BS, I, MO (888-3ADVICE)

About Toners

The purpose of a toner, as the name implies, is to "tone" the skin. This means helping to close down the pores after they've been opened by cleansing. When pores are closed, a smooth, tight surface is created. Ideally, a toner should adjust the pH of the skin so that the protective acid mantle is replaced. In this way, the skin is protected from the environment as well as from makeup, which may be applied over a toner.

My favorite all-purpose toner for every skin type, including acne, used to be pure aloe vera extract. As I mentioned in Chapter 5, aloe vera has myriad qualities that make it suitable as a toner. Its tightening effect closes pores and creates a supersmooth surface that makes makeup application easy and helps makeup to last longer. However, I found daily applications of pure aloe vera to be too drying for any skin type. If you want to make your own toning product, I suggest that you dilute pure aloe vera juice with an equal part of spring water.

I no longer recommend pure aloe vera products by brand name because they can vary so much from one locale to another. However, the guidelines for buying either the gel or the juice are very clear. The product should be between 98 and 100 percent pure aloe, with no oil or water added. The only additives (for product stability) should be ascorbic acid, citric acid, or Irish moss. Again, let me stress that aloe vera in its pure form should only be used medicinally—to heal burns, bites, rashes, and such—and should not be applied to the skin on a daily, ongoing basis. Instead, use aloe in combination with other beneficial ingredients such as herbs, sea water, or floral extracts.

Toner Recommendations

Botanics of California Rosemary Toner	NFS
Earth Science Aloe Vera Complexion Toner & Freshener	NFS
Geremy Rose Strawberry Rose Mist	NFS
Origins Mending Solution	DS
Paul Penders Orange Blossom Yarrow Skin Toner	NFS
Paul Penders Camomile Angelica Skin Toner	NFS
Prescriptives Skin Balancer	DS
Provenance Hydrating Facial Mist	NFS, BS, I, MO (888-3ADVICE)
Zia Cosmetics Sea Tonic Rosewater & Aloe Toner	NFS, MO (800-334-7546)

About Moisturizers

Moisturizers are, without a doubt, the most confusing of all cosmetics. Their purpose is to help skin hold its natural moisture. The original American moisturizers available in the 1940s attempted to seal the skin to prevent moisture from escaping. If they worked at all, it was by protecting skin from the damaging effects of the elements. Unfortunately, continued use eventually caused dryness and other problems, such as clogged pores, blackheads, and slackness of the skin. It's interesting to note, however, that the only women who even thought of using moisturizers back then were those well over 40.

Today, cosmetics companies would have us believe that everyone needs a moisturizer, regardless of age or skin type. This is just not so. A basic moisturizer is needed only by those whose skin lacks sufficient moisture. If your skin type is dry, you should use a moisturizer regardless of your age. Another function of moisturizers, which may be apparent to the naked eye, is to "plump up" the skin, making fine lines less noticeable. In actuality, this is a visual result of the skin holding moisture. For this reason I recommend that most women over 35 with normal skin types use a moisturizer.

Unfortunately, finding a "good moisturizer" can be quite difficult. Cosmetics companies make a wide range of so-called moisturizing products, but their original function—helping the skin hold moisture—seems to have been totally lost. Basic, all-purpose products hardly exist any longer. Instead we have day creams, night creams, throat creams, hydrating formulas, moisture balance formulas, enriching creams, and so forth. A good moisturizer may be used day and/or night on any area of the face and neck. It is not necessary to buy three or four basic moisture creams. In fact, I am absolutely opposed to using thick, greasy creams on the face at night.

For a moisturizer to help the skin hold water, it must contain a humectant—a compound that draws moisture from the air. Some of the most commonly used humectants are glycerin, squalane, hyaluronic acid, jojoba oil, lactic acid, and urea. There is an ongoing dispute among skin-care specialists as to whether a humectant can also draw moisture from the skin. To the best of my knowledge and according to most cosmetics chemists, this can happen only when there is an insufficient source of moisture in a product or available from the atmosphere—that is, in very dry, arid climates or on airplanes. A humectant should never compose more than 20 percent of a product, and the product should contain approximately twice as much water as humectant. If a humectant is listed among the first few ingredients on a label, it is probably too primary in the product.

Most moisturizers are either mineral oil–based, water-based, or natural oil–based. I prefer the latter because they usually contain fewer chemicals or benign chemicals and do the job without causing problems. They also penetrate rather than just sit on the skin. Many of them also cost less than their mineral oil–based counterparts. I believe most commercial moisturizers are grossly overpriced. Their cost has more to do with their expensive packaging and advertising campaigns than with the price of their ingredients. Unless a cream has significant amounts of plant, sea, or herbal extracts, or rich natural oils, essential oils, and vitamins, there is no justification for high cost.

Some other ingredients found in moisturizers are just as bad as mineral oil. A popular one to avoid is petrolatum, which is simply a thicker version of mineral oil. Beeswax, when used as the main ingredient in a product, is too thick and heavy for all but very dry skins. There are also various grades of beeswax; the more highly refined ones are much more acceptable to the skin. Lanolin can be a good ingredient in a moisture cream because it is one of the oils most like that produced by the human body (sebum). However, some people are allergic to lanolin. In recent years, more tolerable forms of lanolin, such as acetylated lanolin or lanolin alcohol, are being used, and usually these are well tolerated by everyone. It is also interesting to know that lanolin is extracted from the wool of sheep and does not cause harm to the animal.

Two chemicals that are difficult to avoid in mass-market moisturizers are Carbomer 934, a thickener that can cause eye irritation, and isopropyl myristate, an emollient that may cause irritation and clog pores. Some people are not sensitive to either of these ingredients, so it is difficult to make a blanket statement about avoiding them. Also, in the case of the latter, over 5 percent must be present in a solution to cause this type of reaction.

An easy way to tell whether these ingredients affect you is to look closely at moisturizers you may have used in the past. If they caused any of the symptoms I've mentioned, cross them off your list and switch to a "cleaner" product. If you have been using a moisturizer that contains one or more of the sensitizing ingredients, with no reaction and with positive results, that indicates it is not problematic for you, and you may wish to continue using it. I never take people off products that are working for them unless the product is dangerous to their health.

If you're not sure whether a particular moisturizer is working well for you, notice what your skin is like if you don't wear it for a day. If your skin is dry, the moisturizer is just masking that condition. If a moisturizer is doing its job, you should be able to go without it for several days before your skin looks dry.

As you can see, choosing a moisturizer is a difficult area in which to make hard-and-fast rules. I can provide you with guidelines, but you must ultimately decide what is right for you by trial and error. As always, I encourage you to return any products you try that are problematic or simply did not do what they were supposed to.

Oil-Based Moisturizers

Moisturizers that are oil-based are usually made with oils such as safflower, almond, jojoba, rice bran, or avocado. These are light enough to be partially or wholly absorbed by the skin and to act as the skin's natural oils—that is, to help the skin hold moisture. Moisturizers that have coconut oil or cocoa butter as a base should not be used because they are saturated fats, making them too heavy to use on the face. Saturated fats have huge molecules, which make them incapable of penetrating the skin. As I have mentioned before, when oils sit on the surface of the skin they usually cause

Oil-Based Moisturizer Recommendations

Annemarie Borlind LL Bi-Activ Regeneration Day Cream	NFS, MO (800-447-7024)
Botanics of California Linden Flower Moisturizer	NFS
Earth Science Almond-Aloe Light & Silky	NFS
Geremy Rose Karite Butter Cream	NFS
Geremy Rose Santa Ana Cream	NFS
Provenance Oxygenated Cranberry Day Cream with SPF	NFS, BS, I, MO (888-3ADVICE)
Provenance Betahydroxy Cranberry Night Cream	(see above)
Weleda Iris Moisturizing Cream	NFS
Zia Cosmetics Nourishing Cream	NFS, MO (800-334-7546)
Zia Cosmetics Everyday Moisturizer	(see above)

Silicone-Based Moisturizers

Several years ago, manufacturers began to replace occlusive oils such as mineral oil with lightweight silicone derivatives such as dimethicone and cyclomethicone. These benign chemicals have the look and feel of oils but do not clog pores, making them better for use by most skin types. However, if you want a truly oil-free product, you should not use products containing significant amounts of these ingredients, because they can look and feel greasy on the skin. Test the product on the inside of your arm to see how it looks and feels.

Silicone-Based Moisturizer Recommendations

Origins Fine Tuner	DS
Prescriptives Oil Free Skin Renewer Lotion	DS
Prescriptives Multi Moisture	DS
Prescriptives Comfort Cream	DS
M.A.C. Moisture Regulating Emulsion	DS

Gel-Based Moisturizers

There are a few moisturizing gels that I highly recommend because of their ability to heal and calm the skin. This type of product is perfect for oily or combination skin because it is oil-free. If oily skin is seriously dehydrated, a treatment oil composed of specific hydrating essential oils should be used for 10 to 14 days to correct the condition. Then a gel-based moisturizer may be used on a daily basis to help maintain hydration and protect and heal the skin.

Gel-Based (Oil-Free) Moisturizer Recommendations

Aqualin	NFS
Company Z Sleek Cheeks Greaseless Face Lotion	NFS, BS, MO, I (888-3ADVICE)
Geremy Rose Royal Papaya Enzyme Gel	NFS
Primavera Immortelle Face Gel	NFS
Zia Cosmetics Herbal Moisture Gel	NFS, MO (800-334-7546)

About Liposome and Oxygenated Products

Products containing liposomes (explained in Chapter 1) supply a deep, time-released source of moisture to the skin. It is difficult to prescribe their usage on a general basis, as skin-care needs vary so much from one person to another. If you are over age 45, however, you probably need to use either a liposome or oxygenating product once or twice a day, since aging skin loses its natural ability to retain moisture. These products should be used under or in place of your regular moisturizer. Many may also be used around the eyes and on the neck, chest, and hands.

Liposome and Oxygenated Product Recommendations

Annemarie Borlind LL
Bi-Aktiv Liposome Emulsion   NFS, MO (800-447-7024)

Provenance Oxygenated   NFS, BS, I,
Cranberry Day Cream with SPF   MO (888-3ADVICE)

Zia Cosmetics Ziasome
Restorative Moisture Treatment   NFS, MO (800-334-7546)

About Eye-Care Products

The purpose of an eye-care product is to protect and lubricate the delicate skin around the eyes and to help minimize lines. For an eye oil or cream to function properly, *it must be water-soluble and quickly absorbed,* because residue left on the skin will cause eye makeup to smudge and run and will also cause problems for contact-lens wearers. Products of this type have been difficult to find but are becoming increasingly available. A water-soluble eye-care product should be used twice a day, following cleansing.

Choosing the right eye oil or cream can be difficult because cosmetics companies do such a good job of making their eye-care products appear "precious." This is done by packaging the product in a tiny, expensive container and charging a fortune for it. If you read the label, you may discover that the ingredients are identical to those found in another of that company's moisturizing creams.

Most mass-market eye creams have a base of mineral oil, petrolatum, or a combination of both. As you know by now, these are basically the same ingredients—by-products of the petroleum industry (that is, what's left over when crude oil is turned into refined oil). Vaseline is petrolatum, and baby oil is mineral oil. Neither has anything to do with minerals or has any nutritional value. Products with these ingredients can cause eye makeup to smudge; when used at night, they make the eyes swell. This edema is actually intended in some products, because when swelling occurs, tiny lines disappear. The problem is that in a few hours, when the swelling goes down, the lines reappear. The continual stretching and shrinking of the skin eventually break down collagen/elastin fibers, and the skin begins to sag.

Women with very dry, aging skin may actually prefer heavier creams that sit on the surface of the skin, because these products reflect light, helping to minimize the appearance of fine lines. If you like this effect, use the product only during the day since using an oily cream at night will cause puffiness.

Eye Treatment Recommendations
Oil-Based

Annemarie Borlind Eye Wrinkle Cream	NFS, MO (800-447-7024)
Botanics of California Immortelle Eye Cream	NFS
Dr. Hauschka Eye Lid Cream	NFS
Earth Science Azulene Desensitizing Eye Cream	NFS
Geremy Rose Cucumber Eye Cream	NFS
M.A.C. EZR Eye Emulsion Day/Night	DS
Paul Penders Carotene Eye Gelee	NFS
Zia Cosmetics Eye Treatment Oil	NFS, MO (800-334-7546)

Oil-Free

Clarins Eye Contour Gel	DS

| PrimeZyme Enzymatic Eye Cream | NFS, BS, MO, I (888-3ADVICE) |
| Provenance Vitamin A Elixir | NFS, BS, I, MO (888-3ADVICE) |

About Essential Oil Treatments

In Chapter 8, I explained the ability of essential oils to penetrate the skin thoroughly—a quality that places them in a class by themselves. Before you decide which oil or oils may be right for you, it's important to understand the difference between therapeutic and cosmetic formulations. Therapeutic formulas are treatment oils that contain 12 to 30 percent essential oils. They are designed to be used for healing for a short period of time, usually 7 to 14 days, then discontinued. Cosmetic formulations containing 1 to 8 percent essential oils may be used as often as you like. The products recommended here are therapeutic essential oil treatment products.

Essential Oil Treatment Recommendations

Alexandra Avery	NFS
Aroma Vera	NFS
Bindi Essential Oil	NFS
Dr. Hauschka's Facial Skin Oil	NFS
Judith Jackson Renewal Face Essence	DS, NFS
Zia Cosmetics Aromatherapy Treatment Oils	NFS, MO (800-334-7546)
Tisserand Aromatherapy	NFS

About Facial Masks

There are three basic types of facial masks used for three distinct purposes: detoxifying masks for cleansing and purifying the skin, moisturizing masks for hydrating and plumping, and toning masks for firming and tightening. Each type has a different composition and function.

Detoxifying Masks

This type of mask draws impurities from the skin and can have a calming effect on active or problem skin. It can also have a tightening effect on pores. Camphor is one of the best ingredients used to detoxify and to draw impurities from the skin. As an esthetician, I was trained to mix oil of camphor into masks to calm down oily skin and take away redness and swelling caused by the extraction of blemishes during a facial. The mask also contains colloidal sulfur, which is used to calm acne and problem skin. The mask does not contain clay and is therefore not drying to the skin. It may be used as often as three times a week to heal and prevent breakouts and to detoxify and calm down the skin. It may also be used as a "spot treatment" for blemishes by applying it directly to a blemish and leaving it on overnight.

I have also recommended some mud- and clay-based masks that do a good job of detoxifying. Remember not to let the mask dry, or it will dehydrate your skin; spray your face with mineral water while the mud or clay mask is on, to keep it moist.

Detoxifying Mask Recommendations

Desert Essence Jojoba Aloe Vera Facial Mask	NFS
Dr. Hauschka's Face Mask	NFS
Kiehl's Rare Earth Mask	DS, MO
Nature's Gate Facial Mask	NFS
Paul Penders Peppermint Arnica Beauty Mask	NFS
Pierre Cattier's Nature de France French Clay Mask	NFS

Reviva Hawaiian Seaweed Beauty Mask	NFS
Company Z Overnight Sensation	NFS, BS, MO, I (888-3ADVICE)
Zia Cosmetics Camphor Treatment Mask	NFS, MO (800-334-7546)

Moisturizing/Hydrating Masks

This type of mask is formulated without clay. Its purpose is to replenish moisture and oil to the skin; thus, it is recommended for dry skin. Women with normal or combination skin may want to use this type of mask when their skin appears to be dry or dehydrated as a result of weather conditions, hormonal changes, travel, and so forth. It may also be used on laugh lines at the corners of the eyes to help plump up and minimize the lines. American cosmetics companies make dozens of masks, but since they are no more than chemical concoctions, I do not recommend them. Natural cosmetics manufacturers and European manufacturers, on the other hand, produce some quality, natural masks for purposes other than moisturization and hydration, but none met our standards of formulation for those specific functions. Since there is only one product in this category,.your best option would be to make your own moisturizing mask according to one of the recipes listed in Chapter 13.

Moisturizing/Hydrating Mask Recommendations

Zia Cosmetics Super Moisturizing Mask	NFS, MO (800-334-7546)

Toning and Firming Masks

These masks are designed to tighten and tone the skin. They sometimes contain clay, but most often have a base of albumen (egg white). This type of mask is most beneficial for older skin that has begun to lose its elasticity. Usually this type of skin has fine lines and wrinkles and sags slightly. A good firming mask will *temporarily* tighten and firm the skin, making lines, wrinkles, and sagging disappear. However, it is important not to use this type of mask in the delicate eye area, as it can put too much stress on this fine, thin skin. You can make your own firming mask by simply applying slightly beaten egg white to your face, but the effects from this will only last a short time.

Toning and Firming Mask Recommendations

Perfectly Taut Facial Mask	NFS
Zia Cosmetics 15 Minute Face Lift	NFS, MO (800-334-7546)

About Facial Sprays

Facial sprays are refreshing water-based products that may be used as toners, to set makeup, or simply as a pick-me-up during the day. Spray over makeup from an arm's length, then allow to dry. Most are more refreshing than therapeutic, allowing you to choose them according to your personal preference and scent.

Facial Spray Recommendations

Aroma Vera Fleur de Brume	NFS, MO (800-669-9514)
Earth Solutions DermaTone	NFS, MO (800-883-3376)
Essential Elements Aroma-therapy Face and Body Mists	NFS, BS
Provenance Hydrating Facial Mist	NFS, BS, I, MO (888-3ADVICE)
Reviva Rosewater Facial Spray With Aloe, Herbs, and Minerals	NFS

Sleepy Hollow Botanicals
NaPCA Skin Moisture Mist   NFS

Zia Cosmetics Sea Tonic
Aloe Toner   NFS, MO (800-334-7546)

About Makeup and Eye Makeup Removers

Unless you are a professional model or an actress in the habit of using stage makeup, I do not recommend makeup removers. They are designed to dissolve oil-based foundation makeup, and I have never found one that was not mineral oil-based. If you use a water-based foundation, cleansing with your usual cleanser will remove it.

Eye makeup removers are fairly straightforward products whose function is solely to remove eye makeup. Before cosmetics companies began manufacturing this product, most women simply used baby oil, and many still do. Baby oil doesn't irritate the eyes, and it's also inexpensive. It is, however, pure mineral oil with a little fragrance, and once applied, it must be removed with tissues, then washed off with soap and water, neither of which is good for the delicate skin around the eyes. With the exception of the products listed below, most oil-based eye makeup removers are usually mineral oil-based and just as bad as baby oil.

Non-oily eye makeup removers are made by most commercial cosmetics companies and often cause eye irritation. Listed below are the ones that work best and are least likely to irritate.

Eye Makeup Remover Recommendations
Oil-Based

Paul Penders Natural Eye
Makeup Remover   NFS

Zia Cosmetics Eye
Treatment Oil   NFS, MO (800-334-7546)

Oil-Free

Almay Hypo-Allergenic Non-Oily Eye Makeup Remover	P
Annemarie Borlind Liquid Eye Makeup Remover	NFS, MO (800-447-7024)
Clarins Eye Makeup Remover Lotion	DS
Kelemata Eye Makeup Remover	DS
Orjene Lipstick and Eye Makeup Remover	NFS
Prescriptives Eye Makeup Remover	DS
Reviva Eye Makeup Remover Gel	NFS
M.A.C. Eye Makeup Remover	DS

Problem Skin Products

Problem Skin Cleansers

Cleansers for problem skin must be oil-free and preferably not be detergent- or soap-based, because these strip the skin of oils and fool it into producing more oil.

Problem Skin Cleanser Recommendations

Aqualin Cleanser	NFS
Cleanzyme	NFS, MO (800-800-0905)
PrimeZyme Oxygenated Papaya Cleanser	NFS, BS, MO, I (888-3ADVICE)
Provenance Cranberry Facial Cleanser	NFS, BS, I, MO (888-323-8423)

Zia Cosmetics Fresh Cleansing
Gel   (see above)

Problem Skin Toners

Toners help close down pores that have been opened by cleansing, thus creating a smooth, tight surface. Ideally, a toner should adjust the pH of the skin so that the protective acid mantle is replaced.

Problem Skin Toner Recommendations

Botanics of California Rosemary Toner	NFS
Clarins Toning Lotion	DS
Earth Science Aloe Vera Complexion Toner & Freshener	NFS
Geremy Rose Tea Mist Toner	NFS
Origins Managing Solution	DS
Paul Penders Peppermint Witch Hazel Skin Toner	NFS
Zia Cosmetics Sea Tonic Aloe Toner	NFS, MO (800-334-7546)

Astringents

The purpose of an astringent is to absorb excess oil, which acts as a breeding ground for bacteria, and to kill the bacteria. Most astringents contain one or more antiseptics in the form of alcohol, witch hazel, or citrus extracts. These should be primary (listed among the first four on the list of ingredients), or the product won't be effective. Many essential oils are also natural bactericides and antiseptics and need only be included in very small amounts of the solution to be effective. An astringent may also contain camphor or menthol, which can be irritating if high amounts are present.

If you enjoy concocting your own cosmetics, a good astringent can be made by mixing together, in a glass jar, the following ingredients: four ounces of witch hazel; four ounces of aloe vera juice; and one-half teaspoon of alum. Due to its lack of preservatives, this mixture should be kept in the refrigerator. For convenience, a small bottle may be kept in the bathroom and refilled once a week.

Astringent Recommendations

Annemarie Borlind U Series Herbal Facial Toner	NFS, MO (800-447-7024)
Company Z Astringent Facial Spritz	NFS, BS, I, MO (888-3ADVICE)
Dickenson's Witch Hazel	P
Dr. Hauschka's Face Lotion "Special"	NFS
Earth Science Clarifying Herbal Astringent	NFS
Reviva Lotion Au Camphor	NFS
M.A.C. Phyto-Astringent Purifying Toner	DS

Problem Skin Moisturizers

Use only oil-free moisturizers, the most beneficial of which is a gel that will protect and regenerate without adding oil or clogging pores. This type of product may be used on all areas of the face, neck, and chest, under makeup and at night before bed. If you have dryness around the eyes, you may use either a liposome or oil-based eye treatment product in this area only.

Problem Skin Moisturizer Recommendations

Aqualin Light	NFS
Company Z Greaseless Face Lotion	NFS, BS, MO, I (888-3ADVICE)
Geremy Rose Royal Enzyme Gel	NFS

Zia Cosmetics Herbal
Moisture Gel   NFS, MO (800-334-7546)

Problem Skin Masks and Treatment Products

For problem skin, you will most likely want to use a
detoxifying mask, as described in the section on masks above.
The treatment products recommended below will help with
breakouts, inflammation, and such. Be sure to read the instructions and follow them carefully. Overuse of treatment
products can cause a variety of skin problems, from whiteheads to irritation. Spot treatments are to be used on pimples
only. Again, follow instructions for each product.

Problem Skin Mask Recommendations

Company Z Cool & Calm   NFS, BS, MO, I (888-3ADVICE
Soothing Facial Mask   or educatedbeauty.com)

Desert Essence Jojoba
Aloe Vera Facial Mask   NFS

Dr. Haushka's Face Mask   NFS

Kiehl's Rare Earth Mask   DS, MO (800-543-4571)

Paul Penders Peppermint
Arnica Beauty Mask   NFS

Pierre Cattier's Clay Mask   NFS

Reviva Hawaiian Seaweed
Beauty Mask   NFS

Borghese Terme de
Monticatini Fango   DS

Zia Cosmetics Camphor
Treatment Mask   NFS, MO (800-334-7546)

Problem Skin Treatment Recommendations

Company Z Overnight   NFS, BS, MO, I (888-3ADVICE
Sensation   or educatedbeauty.com)

Earth Solutions Dermalive   NFS, MO (800-883-3376)

Moiteur   MO (800-257-1241)

Problem Skin Spot Treatment Recommendations

Company Z Zit Styx	NFS, BS, MO, I (888-3ADVICE or educatedbeauty.com)
Desert Essence Australian Tea Tree Oil	NFS
Prescriptives Anti Blemish	DS
Samuel Parr Aromatherapy Pen	DS, NFS, MO (800-448-0800)
Linda Sy Acne Cover Lotion	MO (in California, call 800-232-DERM; outside California, call 800-422-DERM)
Primavera Tea Tree Treatment Gel	NFS
Zia Cosmetics Camphor Treatment Mask	NFS, MO (800-334-7546)

Makeup Products

Foundation Recommendations
Oil-Based

Adriene Arpel Liquid Powder	DS
Aveda Equilibrium Fluid Foundation	S, BS, MO (800-328-0849)
Borghese Hydro-Minerali Natural Finish Makeup	DS
Borghese Molto Bella Liquid Powder Makeup with Sunscreen	DS
Christian Dior Teint Poudre Dual Powder Foundation	DS
Clinique Sensitive Skin Makeup SPF 15	DS
Estee Lauder Fresh Air Makeup	DS
Estee Lauder Lucidity Light-Diffusing SPF 9	DS

Paul Penders Natural Oil-Based Makeup	NFS
Paul Penders Water Base Makeup Cream Foundation	NFS
Prescriptives Soft Matte Makeup	DS
Reviva Liquid Foundation	NFS
Rachael Perry Bee Pollen/Jojoba Nutrient Makeup	NFS

Oil-Free

Almay Fresh Look Oil-Free Makeup	P
Linda Sy Oil-Free Liquid Makeup SPF 15	MO (in California, call 800-232-DERM; outside California, call 800-422-DERM)
Prescriptives Exact Color Makeup 100% Oil-Free, SPF 15	DS
Clinique Pore Minimizer Makeup	DS
M.A.C. Matte Finish Foundation	DS
M.A.C. Satin Finish Foundation	DS
Zia Cosmetics Oil-Free Foundation SPF 18	NFS, MO (800-334-7546)

Face Powder Recommendations

Annemarie Borlind Translucent Powder Compact	NFS, MO (800-447-7024)
Ellegance Sheer Tones	NFS, MO (800-442-3936)
For Seasons Base Basics	MO (408-395-3386)

M.A.C. Pressed Powder Compact	DS
Origins Loose Powder	DS
Paul Penders Translucent Powder	NFS
Real Purity Pressed Powder	MO (800-253-1694)
Sam Fong's Rice Powder	BS
Zia Cosmetics Natural Translucent Face Powders	NFS, MO (800-334-7546)

Blush Recommendations

Annemarie Borlind Powder Rouge	NFS, MO (800-447-7024)
Clinique Beyond Blusher Oil-Free Everywhere Color	DS
Clinique Cheek Base	DS
Elegance Vibrance Blusher	NFS, MO (800-442-3936)
For Seasons	MO (408-395-3386)
M.A.C. MACnificent Powder Blush	DS
Origins Brush On Color	DS
Paul Penders Loose Powder Blusher	NFS
Real Purity Powder Blush	MO
Zia Cosmetics Bronzing Powder	NFS, MO (800-334-7546)

Undereye Concealer Recommendations

Borgese	DS
Origins Concealer	DS
Prescriptives	DS

Eyeliner Recommendations

Logona Eyeliners	NFS
M.A.C. Cream Liners	DS

Eye Shadow Recommendations

Clinique Eye Treats	DS
Estee Lauder Eye Coloring	DS
Prescriptives Eye Shadow Pencils	DS
Prescriptives Eye Shadow Powders	DS
Reviva Eye Shadows	NFS
Paul Penders Eye Shadow	NFS
M.A.C. Eye Shadow	DS

Mascara Recommendations

Arbonne Mascara	CR (800-ARBONNE)
Estee Lauder Moisture Binding Formula Mascara	DS
Kelemata Mascara	DS
M.A.C. Mascara	DS
Paul Penders Mascara	NFS
Reviva Liquid Mascara	NFS
Revlon Sheer Tint	P

Lip Pencil Recommendations

Logona Lip Pencil	DS
M.A.C. Lip Pencil	DS

Lipstick Recommendations

Paul Penders	NFS
Terra Verde	NFS
Borlind of Germany	NFS

Orjene	NFS
M.A.C.	DS
Origins	DS
Prescriptives	DS
Real Purity	MO (800-253-1694)
Zia Cosmetics Natural Translucent Face Powder	NFS

Body-Care Products

About Soaps and Cleansers

Soap dries the skin, and I don't believe it is necessary to use it all over the body on a daily basis. My recommendation is to use soap only where it is needed and to use a non-soap- or non-detergent-based cleanser with a loofah in other areas. If you must use soap, avoid Ivory soap and deodorant soaps because they leave a film on the surface of the skin and are the most drying. Glycerin soaps, or those containing emollients, are the least drying. Soaps made from pure olive oil are another excellent choice and are easy to find in health food stores or cosmetics/bath shops. In general, liquid body cleansers are preferable to soaps, but don't use ones that contain sodium laureth sulfate, which can strip the body's natural oils.

Body Cleanser Recommendations

Alba Botanica Body Baths	NFS
Annemarie Borlind Body Wash Lotion	NFS, MO (800-447-7024)
Aroma Vera Home Spa System Aromatic Bath & Shower Gel	NFS, MO (800-669-9514)
Company Z Dynamic Duo Face & Body Wash	I (educatedbeauty.com)
Paul Penders Shower Gel	NFS
Zia Cosmetics Absolutely Pure Aloe & Citrus Wash	NFS, MO ((800-334-7546)

About Body Moisturizers

A good body moisturizer is an absolute necessity for most of us past age 35. Daily body moisturizing can be accomplished with either body lotions, alphahydroxy acid lotions and gels, or body oils. You can choose whatever feels best to your skin and feel free to alternate them regularly.

Body Lotions

A body lotion is not a product to be stingy with; it should be applied liberally, twice a day. Since the skin on the rest of your body isn't nearly as sensitive or delicate as that on the face and neck, body lotions that contain mineral oil, petrolatum, and coconut oil are okay to use. I still prefer non-mineral-oil products, however, which are readily available. People with very dry skin may find a mineral oil–based product preferable to a natural oil–based one, because the former are more occlusive and less expensive. If you like a shiny look on your bare legs in the summer, this type of product is for you! There is very little difference between most mineral oil-based lotions. You may choose the fragrance, price, or packaging you like best. Just remember that there is no therapeutic value to these products. They work only while they are on your skin by masking the symptoms of dryness.

In order for a lotion to *heal* dry skin, it must contain penetrating oils or water-binding ingredients such as lecithin, aloe vera, hyaluronic acid, shea (karite) butter, vitamins, or essential oils. Continued use of this type of product actually helps to repair dry skin. A health food store is the place to shop if you would prefer to use a natural oil–based body lotion. Many of these contain healing ingredients such as aloe vera and herbal and plant extracts.

Body Lotion Recommendations

Alba Botanica Very Emollient
Body Lotion   NFS

Annemarie Borlind Body Balm	NFS, MO (800-447-7024)
Autumn Harp Body Lotion	NFS
Body Love's Aromalotion	NFS
Botanee Hand & Body Lotion with Karite Nut Butter	NFS
Dr. Hauschka's Body Milk	NFS
Eucerin Cream or Lotion	P
Geremy Rose Sweet Almond Body Creme	NFS
Home Health Almond Glow Skin Lotion	NFS
Mountain Ocean Skin Trip	NFS
Nature's Gate Moisturizing Lotion with Papaya	NFS
Nature's Gate Skin Therapy	NFS
Nutriderm Lotion	P
Origins Steady Drencher	DS
Paul Penders Calming Flower Body Lotion	NFS
Paul Penders Oriental Flower Body Lotion	NFS
Primavera Body Lotion Relaxing/Invigorating	NFS
Provenance Cranberry Lotion for the Body	NFS, BS, I, MO (see above)
Reviva Seaweed Body Treatment Lotion	NFS
Zia Cosmetics Essential Body Moisturizer	NFS, MO (800-334-7546)

Alphahydroxy-Acid Body Lotions and Gels

AHA body lotions and gels contain up to 10 percent alphahydroxy acid. They help to slough off dead skin and repair the signs of photoaging, such as uneven skin color and rough texture.

Alphahydroxy-Acid Body Lotion
and Gel Recommendations

Lachydrin	RX
Paul Penders Herbal Citrus Exfoliant for the Body	NFS

Body Oils

Body oils are light, vegetable-based oils that also sometimes contain essential oils. They are designed to be applied to skin that is wet from a shower or bath, as they penetrate the skin along with the water. If you have a favorite body lotion, you may want to use it over a body oil to really seal in moisture.

Body Oil Recommendations

Aroma Vera Body Oils	NFS, MO (800-669-9514)
Aveda Calming or Energizing Nutrients	S, BS, MO (800-328-0849)
Bindi Herbal Massage & Body Oil	NFS
Bindi Herbal Body Treatment Blend	NFS
Body Love's Aromalotion	NFS
Desert Essence Aromatherapy Body Oil Collection	NFS

Dr. Hauschka's Body Oil Blackthorn Composition	NFS
Earth Science Concentrated Apricot Body & Facial Oil	NFS
Jurlique Body Care Oil	DS
Natural Hawaiian Skin Care's Kukui Nut Oil	NFS
Nature's Acres Body Oils	MO (800-499-4372)
Neutrogena Body Oil	P
Olbas Sport Swiss Massage & Vitamin Skin Oil	NFS
Orjene Sweet Almond Oil	NFS
Sea Enzyme Normalizing Seaweed Body Oil	NFS
Weleda Citrus Body Oil	NFS

About Bath Oils

Natural bath oils are available in health food stores and specialty bath shops. Many of these products are "sulfonated" to allow them to dissolve in water rather than simply floating on the surface. All of the bath oils recommended are formulated with essential oils that have a powerful effect on the body. You can also create your own treatment baths by adding one to three drops of essential oil to bathwater.

Bath Oil Recommendations

Alexandra Avery Bath Blend	NFS
Aroma Vera Bath Oils	NFS, MO (800-669-9514)
Baudelair Bath Oil	NFS
Body Love's Lemon Ginger Joy Aroma Beads	NFS

Crystal Essence Bath Oils	NFS
Dr. Hauschka's Lemon & Lavender Bath	NFS
Kneipp Bath Oils	NFS
Origins Bath Oil	DS
Paul Penders Creamy Bath Oil	NFS
Primavera Relaxing Bath and Invigorating Bath Oil	NFS
Santa Fe Bath Oils	MO (505-473-1717)
Weleda Bath Oils	NFS
Quan Yin Essentials Massage Oil	NFS, MO (707-431-0529)

Bath Salt/Product Recommendations

Alexandra Avery Bath Blend	NFS
Aroma Vera Aromatic Bath Salts	NFS, MO (800-669-9514)
Chatoyant Pearl Lavender Bath Potpourri	NFS
Dr. Singha's Mustard Bath	NFS, MO (512-444-2862)
Essential Elements Bath Salts	NFS
Jericho Dead Sea Bath Salts	NFS
Masada Dead Sea Bath Salts	NFS
Nature's Acres Bath Salts	MO (800-499-4372)

About Body Powders

One great way to keep the skin feeling soft and dry especially during the summer months is with a body powder. In the past I have been reluctant to recommend body powders because the primary ingredient is usually talc (an inferior absorbent that is also harmful to the lungs when inhaled). Since the publication of my last book, I have found a few cornstarch-based formulations that I am happy to recommend here.

Body Powder Recommendations

Alexandra Avery Purely Natural Moon Silk Body Powder	NFS
Aura Cacia Natural Body Powders	NFS
Autumn Harp Talc Free Baby Powder	NFS
Burt's Bees Green Goddess Dusting Powder	NFS
Kama Sutra Honey Dust	NFS

About Body Exfoliating Products

Loofahs are sold in pharmacies, health food stores, department stores, and bath shops, in their original long shape, which ranges from 10 to 36 inches; the longer ones make good back brushes. Loofahs are also available in smaller, hand-sized pieces or sewn together with terry cloth to make a "loofah mitt." All types and sizes are equally effective. Choose the one that is best suited to your needs.

Many health food stores and bath shops offer natural-bristle "dry" brushes. One of my favorites is the old-fashioned back brush designed to reach all the way down your back. Its long wooden handle is detachable; the boar-bristle brush head has a cloth handle that makes it easy to hold.

Agave is a desert cactus whose fibers are woven into a rough cloth. Used as a washcloth, it is rough enough to exfoliate even the most stubborn skin cells. Other good scrubbers are made of nylon and are available through beauty supply stores.

Body Exfoliating Product Recommendations

Amazing Grains Facial/Body Cleanser	NFS
Desert Essence Jojoba Facial Scrub	NFS
Reviva Honey-Almond Scrub	NFS
Alba Botanica Gentle Body Smoother	NFS
Aroma Vera Aromatic Cleansing Scrub	NFS, MO (800-669-9514)
Aroma Vera Aromatic Shower Gel Exfolient	(see above)

Body Brushes/Loofahs Recommendations

Smith & Hawken Agave Scrub Cloth	NFS, MO (415-383-2000)
Smith & Hawken Palm Fiber Massage Brush	(see above)
Flower Massage	P

About Natural Fragrances

Natural fragrances are perfumes made with essential oils rather than artificial fragrance. They are often more appropriate for people with sensitive skin who are allergic to artificial fragrance. They can be used instead of perfume to scent an unscented body lotion or oil. Try putting a few drops in bathwater. Some essential oils can be photosensitizing, however, and should not be applied to the nape of the neck or other sun-exposed areas as they may cause hyperpigmentation (skin discoloration).

Natural Fragrance Recommendations

Santa Fe Perfumes	MO (505-473-1717)
L'Artisan Parfumeur	MO (800-840-6835)

Neal's Yard Aromatic
Cologne   DS, NFS, MO (800-570-3775)

About Hand-Care Products

Since hands are one of the first places to show signs of aging and since they are always exposed to the elements as well as to detergents and chemicals, it is important to protect them on a daily basis. Many anti-aging products for the face can also be used on the hands—AHA and BHA creams, enzyme creams, hydrating masks, antioxidant creams, and cellular renewal moisturizers. In the daytime, use a moisturizing sunblock with an SPF 15 or higher instead of regular hand lotion and reapply it often. At night, use the richest hand cream you can find and massage it into your cuticles to keep them supple.

Hand-Care Product Recommendations

Annemarie Borlind Hand Balm	NFS, MO (800-447-7024)
Dr. Hauschka's Hand Creme	NFS
Logona Hand Cream	NFS
Nature's Gate Skin Therapy	NFS
Origins Handle with Care	DS
Paul Penders Hand Creme	NFS
Provenance Oxygenated Cranberry Moisturizer with SPF	NFS, BS, MO, I (888-3ADVICE)
Primavera May Blossom Hand and Nail Repair	NFS
Speick Hand Cream	NFS
Weleda Rose Petal Hand Cream	NFS

About Foot Care

The feet are often the most ignored parts of the body, and the neglect shows in dryness, roughness, and calluses. We all know how good it feels to have our feet massaged, so I suggest that you do it yourself! Rub a good quality moisturizer into your feet every night as you massage them. If you have tough, rough spots, rub them with a pumice stone or with some form of scrubber while in the bath or shower.

Foot-Care Product Recommendations

Aquasole Cushioned Insoles	MO (800-626-7888)
Arbonne Herbal Foot Care	CR, MO (800-ARBONNE)
Hauschka Sage Foot Bath	NFS
Hauschka Rosemary Lotion	NFS
Gilden Tree Footscrubber & Massage Oil	NFS
Weleda Citrus Foot Cream	NFS

Sun-Care Products

Substances that protect the skin from the sun's damaging rays may be the most important anti-aging products you use. There are now hundreds of these products available in a variety of formulations. Almost all the sunblocks on the market are chemical blocks that use chemicals such as TEA-salicylate, benzophenone 3 or 4, and octyl methoxycinnamate as active ingredients.

Recently, a new type of sunblock using a physical sunblocking ingredient called micronized titanium dioxide has come on the market. Despite its chemical-sounding name, titanium dioxide is a naturally occurring mineral. It acts as a broad-spectrum sunblock, protecting the skin by reflecting both UVA and UVB rays away from the body.

In order for a sun-blocking product to be issued an SPF (sun protection factor) number, it must be tested according to guidelines recommended by the Federal Drug Administration. Sunblocks with SPF numbers are considered to be over-the-counter drugs and must strictly comply with FDA labeling laws by listing their active (sun-blocking) ingredients. The purpose for this is consumer protection, and it is very important in this type of product, especially since so many people are allergic to PABA and its derivative Padimate-O. For your protection, do not purchase any product that makes an SPF claim without listing by name the specific sun-blocking ingredients it contains.

Although the higher the SPF number, the higher the protection, this also means the higher the chance of irritation. So only use an SPF higher than 17 when it is needed. The exception to this rule is the use of physical blocks. These may have an SPF as high as 40 without any skin irritation, because the sun-blocking ingredient is physical rather than chemical. As I explained in Chapter 3, there is no approved rating system for UVA protection, which means that the SPF on a product only reflects the protection you get against UVB rays. Until a rating system for UVA rays is approved by the FDA, the only way to know what UVA protection a product affords is to contact the manufacturer to find out the percentage of UVA blocker the product contains and how much of the UVA spectrum it blocks.

I have not included any products that are mineral oil–based because there are so many natural oil–based sunblocks available that won't clog pores or dehydrate the skin. Sunblocks with mineral oil may be used only by people with dry skin. Other skin types should use oil-free products and should avoid those with a high percentage of alcohol, which can be drying to the skin. Some products are fine for the body but not suitable for use on the face, because they contain primary ingredients such as coconut oil or high amounts of fragrance and other potentially sensitizing ingredients. These products are designated with an asterisk (*).

Oil-Free Sunblocks

The following sunblock is the only true oil-free product I know of; it contains no oils of any kind nor silicone derivatives (cyclomethicone, dimethicone). These silicone ingredients, found in other products labeled "oil-free," leave a greasy residue on the surface of the skin.

Zia Cosmetics Oil-Free
FaceBlock SPF 16   NFS, MO (800-334-7546)

Oil-Free Silicone-Based Sunblocks for Face and Body

The following sunblocks are oil-free yet contain silicone derivatives (cyclomethicone, dimethicone), which leave an oily residue on the surface of the skin. These sunblocks may be used by those with normal and combination skin.

Almay SPF 30+ Waterproof
Sunblock   P

Alo Sun Fashion Tan Oil-Free
Sunblock Spray SPF 15   P

*Bullfrog SPF 18 Lotion, 36 Gel   P

DermAesthetics Ultra Sunblock
SPF 25   MO (Dermatologic
                                    Specialty Products,
                                    P.O. Box 83, Livingston,
                                    NJ 07039)

Estee Lauder Sun Oil-Free
Sunspray SPF 15   DS

Nature's Gate Natural Suncare
Sports Dry Lotion SPF 15   NFS

Neutrogena No-Stick Sunscreen
SPF 30   P

Orjene Oil-Free Sunscreen Spray SPF 14	NFS
Prescriptives SPF 15 Mist	DS

Oil-Based Sunblocks for Face and Body

The following sunblocks are appropriate for use on the face as well as the body. I recommend using an oil-based sunblock for dry and aging skin.

Alba Botanica Day-One Sun Care Lotion SPF 16	NFS
Almay Fragrance-Free Suncare Waterproof Moisturizing Lotion SPF 15 and 20	P
Aloe Up Suncare Lotion 20	P, NFS
Clarins Sun Block Total Protection SPF 25	DS
Clinique Face Zone Sun Block SPF 15	DS
Clinique Total Cover Sun Block SPF 30	DS
Dura Screen All Day Sunscreen SPF 15	P
Dura Screen Waterproof Sunscreen Lotion	P
Dura Screen SPF 30	P
Jason's Natural Duck Oil Sunblock SPF 18	NFS
Jason's SunBrella's Family Sunscreen SPF 30+	NFS
Jason's SunBrella's Moisturizing Aloe Vera Sunscreen SPF 16 and 26	NFS

Lily of the Desert Skin Saver
SPF 16 and 40   NFS

Linda Sy Optimal Light
Textured Sunscreen Lotion
SPF 15   MO (in California, call
                                   1-800-232-DERM;
                                   outside California, call
                                   1-800-422-DERM)

Mountain Ocean SPF 15   NFS

Nature's Gate Natural Suncare
Suntan Lotion SPF 15 and 30   NFS

*Rachel Perry Aloe Suma All
Seasons Sunblock SPF 15   NFS

*Rachel Perry Aloe Suma
Advanced Treatment Sunblock
SPF 24   NFS

Physical Sunblocks

Because the physical block is so effective, I have also
included products with lower SPFs. Some leave a faint white
film on the skin, especially when the skin is wet. The
Provenance product leaves no film.

*Aloe Up Chemical Free
Sunscreen SPF 30   P, NFS

Banana Boat Natural Chemical
Free Sunblock SPF 15 and 25   P

*Clinique Special Defense Sun
Block SPF 25   DS

Linda Sy Non-Chemical
Sunscreen SPF 16   (see order info above)

Natural Tanning Formula
Natural Protection SPF 15 and 25   MO (800-848-7623)

Neutrogena Chemical-Free Sunblocker SPF 17	P
*Origin's Let the Sun Shine SPF 14 and 21	DS
Orjene Chemical Free Sunscreen Lotion SPF 14	NFS
Provenance Oxygenated Cranberry Day Cream with SPF	NFS, BS, I, MO (888-3ADVICE)

Sunsticks

Sunsticks are essentially oil-based sunblocks in stick form. You might try these as a handy alternative to lotions or creams. The rule of thumb to follow: If it contains mineral oil or petrolatum, use it on the lips, ears, and body only; if it doesn't, you can use it all over, as you would any sunblock.

*Bullfrog Sunblock Stick SPF 18	P
Clarins Sunblock Stick SPF 19	DS
Neutrogena Sunblock Stick SPF 25	P
Prescriptives Advanced Sun Protection SPF 30 Sunstick	DS

Lip Blocks

It is important to remember that the lips are just as vulnerable to sun damage as the rest of your face. For those susceptible to herpes simplex I (cold sores), it is vital to use an SPF 15 or higher lip block at all times, as ultraviolet light triggers this condition. Most lipsticks do not provide adequate sun protection. Use one of the lip blocks everyday under, or instead of, your regular lipstick.

Almay's All-Season Moisture Stick #15	P
Aloe Up Lip Ice SPF 15	P, NFS
Aloe Up Weatherproof Lip Protector	(see above)
Banana Boat Aloe Vera Lip Balm SPF 21	P
Chap Stick Ultra Sunscreen #15	P
Jason's SunBrella's Lip Guard SPF 18	NFS
Lily of the Desert SPF 16	NFS
Linda Sy Lip Balm SPF 15	MO (see order info above)
Mountain Ocean Lip Trip SPF 15	NFS
*Nature's Gate Lip Balm SPF 15	NFS
Neutrogena Lip Moisturizer SPF 15	P
Prescriptives #15 Lip Shield	DS
Un-Petroleum Lip Balm SPF 18	NFS

Hand Cream with Sunblock

Any of the rich, oil-based sunblocks listed above may be used on the hands as a hand cream. You should keep whatever product you use in your car so that you can apply it as needed. A physical block is best for this purpose since if offers immediate protection, while a chemical block must be applied 20 to 30 minutes prior to exposure before protection can take place.

Moisturizers with Sunblock

Even though good moisturizers with an SPF of 15 or higher are in great demand, there are still very few that are well made. Remember that any of the oil-based sunblocks I recommend for use on the face contain good moisturizing ingredients and may be used as a protective moisturizer.

Earth Science Almond-Aloe Facial Moisturizer SPF 15	NFS
Linda Sy Optimal Moisturizer Sunscreen SPF 15	MO (see order info above)
Nature's Gate Petal Fresh Moisturizer SPF 15	NFS
Neutrogena Moisture SPF 15	P
Prescriptives Outdoor Protection SPF 15 Moisturizer	DS

Makeup with Sunblock

Most foundation makeups, whether liquid or powder, will afford a certain amount of protection from ultraviolet light if they contain iron oxides. (Iron oxides work like titanium oxide to reflect UVA and UVB rays.) There are a few foundations on the market that are specifically designed to block the sun. I recommend wearing one of them in place of your usual foundation makeup on a daily basis during the summer months. The following is a list of different types of makeup that contain a minimum of SPF 15.

Foundation

Clinique Sensitive Skin Makeup SPF 15	DS
Linda Sy Oil-Free Liquid Makeup SPF 15	MO (see order info above)
Prescriptives Exact Color Makeup SPF 15	DS

Zia Cosmetics Oil-Free
Foundation SPF 18   NFS, MO (800-334-7546)

Lipstick
Clinique Sun Buffer Lipstick
SPF 15   DS
Borghese Lip Treatment SPF 15   DS

Concealer
Clinique Eye-Zone Sun Block
SPF 14   DS

Bronzing Products

If you are considering using a bronzing product (a tinted gel that provides an "instant" tan and can be washed off), you have many to choose from. Almost every mass-market cosmetic company now offers a bronzer; since they are all similarly formulated, it is mostly a matter of finding one that is right for you. I suggest you conduct sample patch-tests to find one that best complements your skin's natural color. There are also many bronzing powders to choose from; however, I recommend selecting one that doesn't contain talc.

Bronzing Powder Recommendations
Ellegance Vibrance Blusher   NFS, MO (800-442-3936)
For Seasons Face Powder   BS, S, MO (408-395-3386)
Zia Cosmetics Bronzing
Powder   NFS, MO (800-334-7546)

About Self-Tanning Products

One of the best innovations in skin savers comes in the form of the new "self-tanning" products. These give the look of a natural tan without sun exposure and without harming the skin. In my opinion, they are the only truly safe way to

tan your skin. The "tanning" ingredient is dihydroxyacetone, a keto sugar that reacts with the protein on the surface
of skin to create the look of a tan. Most people will turn the
same color tan that they would normally get from the sun.
The molecules of dihydroxyacetone are too big to penetrate
more than the most superficial layers of skin, making it safe
for anyone to use. The tan fades gradually like a real tan.

Before using one of these products on your face, try it
on your body, as it may fade unevenly. This is not readily
noticed on legs and arms. Self-tanning creams may also contain mineral oil or other undesirable chemicals that can
cause clogged pores or breakouts on the face but won't affect
the rest of the body's skin.

Don't be tempted by "tanning pills" now being adver-
tised in magazines and health food stores. They contain high
amounts of beta-carotene, which causes the skin to turn
orange. Another popular ingredient in such pills is canthax-
anthin, which is not approved as a food additive by the FDA
and may also cause liver damage. There is, however, a
promising new tanning pill that has not yet received FDA
approval. It causes the body to produce melanin as it would
when you get a suntan. If all goes well, it may be available by
1995 or 1996.

I have been gratified to see more and more self-tanning
products on the market because it indicates that people are
trying safer alternatives to tanning. Since I have listed all the
products that perform satisfactorily, you have quite a range
to choose from. Some of the new self-tanning products listed
even contain sunblock.

Almay Fragrance Free Sunless Tanning Lotion	P
Annemarie Borlind Sunless Bronze	NFS
Clarins Self-Tanning Milk SPF 6	DS

Clarins Creme Solaire Anti-Rides Self Tanning Face Cream SPF 15	DS
Clinique Self-Tanning Formula	DS
Estee Lauder Self-Action Tanning Cream	DS
Estee Lauder Super Tan	DS
Hawaiian Tropic Self Tanning Sunblock SPF 15	P
Nature's Gate Natural SunCare Self-Tanning Lotion	NFS
Neutrogena Glow Sunless Tanning Spray	P
Origins Summer Vacation	DS
*Prescriptives Sun Free Tanner	DS
Zia Cosmetics Sans Sun Self-Tanning Creme	NFS, MO (800-334-7546)

Natural Insect Repellants

Many people who spend time outdoors during the summer have asked me about natural insect repellants. Deet, the main ingredient in most commercial bug repellants, is extremely harsh to the skin and smells vile! I am happy to recommend several alternatives that use essential oils instead of deet to repel insects.

Aroma Vera Insect Repellant Oil	NFS, MO (800-669-9514)
Ecosafe Skeeter Off	NFS
Greenban for People & Greenban for People Double Strength	NFS
Lakon Herbals by Gone Bugs	NFS
Mountain Sun Don't Bug Me	NFS

15 Love and Longevity

I have three things to tell you about true love:

1. It exists.

2. You can have it.

3. You may not find it where you think it should be.

My father was one of the sweetest, most loving, and truly kind-hearted human beings I've ever known. He died last year at age 83 while still married to my mother, his wife of 56 years. His last words to her were "You're beautiful."

All of my life I remember him telling me, "There's someone for everyone." You can see for yourself how true that statement is if you begin to notice couples. People may be short, tall, skinny, fat, sloppy, loud, quiet, handsome, homely, or any combination of a hundred descriptions; they may be rich, poor, educated, uneducated, funny, dour, or possess an unlimited number of characteristics and circumstances; but regardless of someone's personality, looks, sexual proclivity, or social status, at some point in their lives most people find others that they can relate to. Many find partners who complement or at least "fit" with their particular needs. Very often two people find each other and seem to be "made for each other." This is what most of us think of as "true love." In truth, it is only one source of what we experience as "true love."

We all have our own personal "pictures" of what we think true love will look like, or should look like. Yet when you begin observing what the reality of that is, it often doesn't resemble what we thought it would. Very often, it appears in a form that we never even considered possible.

I believe the secret to finding your true love is to ready yourself properly so that you can recognize it when it comes along. Sometimes this happens totally unbidden: love at first sight; you know in an instant. How many times have you met someone and felt that you'd met before, even though you knew you hadn't? How many times have you met someone and felt so comfortable within a few minutes of talking with them that you felt as if you'd known them for many years or even all your life? No one really knows what causes this type of phenomenon but it happens to everyone in one way or another, and it may be a sign. If you look closely at what took place in a person's life prior to that moment of "love at first sight," you will most likely see two people who seem to have spent their lives leading up to that moment, preparing themselves unconsciously for each other. Had they met a year or even a month sooner, they might not have been ready.

My mother loves to tell the story of how she and my father met and, although I've heard it many times, each time I still get chills. My mother loved to dance. One Friday night she went to a dance with one of her girlfriends in spite of the fact that she had almost canceled because she was tired. They stayed for awhile and each danced with several young men. Then my mother gave in to her tiredness and put on her hat and coat to leave. Just as she did this, she saw my father walk in the door. She immediately looked at her friend and said, "I'm going to leave before this wise guy asks me to dance." (It's impossible for me to imagine anyone thinking of my father as a "wise guy.") No sooner were the words out of her mouth than my father walked directly over to her and asked her to dance. She always says she had no idea why she said yes. They danced together until the dance was over and, at the end, my father asked for her phone number. At this point, she says, "I never gave my real number to *any* of the boys I danced with, but I gave it to your father and I couldn't figure out why. I said to my friend, 'I gave him my number!'" Eight months later they were married. On their wedding day, my mother was 26 years old; for 1937, that was considered a good candidate to be an old maid. She tells me that she was so choosey about young men that even her own mother used to tell her that if she didn't "settle" for someone soon she'd never get married at all! But she knew that she was looking for something that she hadn't yet found. She couldn't articulate exactly what that was, but knew she'd recognize it when she saw it, and she had been prepared to spend her life as a single woman if she never found it. Fortunately for me, she "saw something" in my father.

Another interesting little piece to this story happened six weeks after their initial meeting. In my mother's words, "One of my girlfriends dragged me in to see this fortune-teller. I'd never done anything like that and neither had she. It was a Russian tearoom, and after we'd drunk our tea, a woman came to our table and read my tea leaves. She looked into the cup and said, 'I see the initials W and E. (These are the first initials of my mother's two brothers.) They are very close to you, but they are being pushed aside by someone whose initials are HK (my father's initials).' At this point I looked at my girlfriend who was sitting there with her mouth hanging open and her eyes wide, like she'd seen a ghost. 'You're going to marry this HK,' the woman said, and I said to my girlfriend, 'Let's get out of here!' "

For me, that story always brings up the question of fate. Are our lives mapped out in some grand plan that is stamped into our DNA at the time of conception? Is that what makes it possible for fortune tellers and astrologers to know our futures? Is that why we sometimes move in directions or make decisions based on intuition rather than fact? And what does all of this have to do with staying youthful into old age? Everything.

First, let's look at what you can do to find your true love. As I mentioned earlier, I believe that the key is to make yourself ready. This means clearing away fear and resistance. Everyone has varying degrees of both, usually as a result of past failure in relationships that can go back as far as early childhood. Working on any "issues" (my least favorite word) that you may have is step number one. This doesn't necessarily mean going into therapy, although if your issues are particularly strong, you may want to deal with them this way. There are numerous workshops and retreats designed for this purpose, some lasting a weekend or two and others taking place over longer periods of time. Reading books or joining a peer group designed to bring things out in the open where they can be more easily understood can both help. Writing your feelings and thoughts out on paper can sometimes be very helpful. Or simply getting together with a friend to share feelings with someone you trust. Once you think you know your feelings more clearly and have confronted your fears concerning relationships, you can begin to focus on what you really want. At this point, I believe that it is more than helpful—it is imperative—to write down on paper a complete description of the person you think you would like to have as your partner. Be as specific as possible in all areas except physical. I think it's better to leave the physical characteristics as a general description. Keep that piece of paper somewhere where you can refer to it often and make any changes that come to your mind. As soon as you've got it just right, tuck it away somewhere safe. From then on, try to spend a few minutes every day picturing yourself with the person you've described. See yourself doing everyday things together like eating dinner, taking walks, or laughing and talking. Most important, imagine how you'll feel in his/her company. You'll notice that the more realistically you can imagine, the more that actual feelings will come into play. You'll begin to feel the way you actually would in real situations with that person. When you do meet that person, you'll know right away because you'll be familiar with your own feelings. If this sounds too far-fetched to you right now, try it anyway. You don't have to believe in it for it to work. You just have to make your imagery as real as you possibly can.

Although my mother had found her true love in 1937, she had several key issues from her youth that she systematically refused to confront because they were too painful. Whenever one of these subjects came into her mind or into a conversation, she would become very upset and within a few minutes simply "put it out of her mind." This inability to deal with her feelings affected the quality of her life. Last month, her usual pattern emerged when one of these topics came into our conversation. But all of a sudden I seemed to understand what was driving her fear, her inability to face the pain and sorrow of these subjects. I said, "Mother, are you afraid that if you really let yourself feel all the sadness you have about this, you'll die?" She thought for a moment and then answered, "Yes. I'm afraid that it will hurt so much I won't be able to go on living." That fear had affected almost every aspect of her life for more than 60 years! When she realized this and allowed herself to feel the emotions she had buried, she wept openly for a long time. She was very sad for the next few days and cried often. Then something happened that was no less than a miracle. My family and I watched my mother transform before our eyes. She laughed more than I had heard her laugh since I was a child, sometimes so hard that it brought tears to her eyes. Her attitude changed from one of basic negativity ("All these wild deer around your house . . . don't you worry about Lyme disease?") to an incredibly positive one ("Can you believe this rain? Maybe we'll see a rainbow!"). Everyone who has seen her recently has made a point of calling me to tell me that she looks *20 years younger*. They all want to know what happened. I believe that what my mother uncovered when she gave up her fear was love. My father was gone, but suddenly my mother found love everywhere: in her great-grandchild, in the beauty of the desert and the mountains, in the small colorful rocks that she collected on her daily walks, and in the company of friends and family. She had held a portion of herself in check, protecting herself, and suddenly she began to really share herself with others; it was exhilarating.

Your true love may not be what you thought you wanted at all. So often our desires are influenced by the desires of others: our family and friends, magazines, television, movies, and especially commercials and ads. On a daily basis, we are bombarded by what others want us to want. It can be very difficult to discern what is truly right for us. Your true love may not even be a person. It may be something you've always wanted to do, somewhere you've always wanted to go, or as simple as a quiet place within yourself that you haven't ever known existed.

What has all this got to do with longevity? Everything. The simple fact is that people who love live longer. In recent years, this has been illustrated by the results of many different studies. One proved that elderly people lived longer, more illness free, and happier lives when they owned pets. Another showed the same result when elders spent several hours each week in the company of children. And the most recent study indicates that people live longer and enjoy a better quality of life when they are in loving relationships, rather than being single. So, what's love got to do with it? Everything!

Did you ever stop to think about the innumerable ways in which love reaches into our lives? As children, we inspire and return unconditional love for our parents and family. When we get a little older, we love our pets, our favorite stuffed animal, and even a favorite "blankie." We learn to love certain foods, games, characters in movies, maybe even the kid next door. We love certain times of the year and times of the day, natural wonders, sunsets, sailboats, and the brilliant color of a tropical flower. I believe it is the feeling we get when we feel "love" that keeps us youthful.

A year and a half ago when my granddaughter was born, I remembered the particular feeling of unconditional love that I had felt when my daughter was an infant. I realized in that first moment of holding tiny Caili in my arms, when she was less than one day old, that I hadn't felt that particular feeling for more than 20 years. It was a blissful joy that bubbled up from somewhere deep within me and brought with it elation. What I now believe is that we can experience that same feeling via many different routes, simply by being open to the possibility that it can happen. Since that moment when I first held Caili in my arms, I have experienced very similar feelings in many different situations: with the man I love, hiking one mile straight up to a meadow 9000 feet above the valley floor in Colorado, watching the sun set over the ocean, sitting in meditation, seeing a stand of aspens shimmering in the sunlight, and after singing for a small group of close friends. It seems that the more I recognize and acknowledge this feeling, the more I feel it. And it seems to bring several things along with it, not the least of which is a sense of well-being that shows. Over the past year and a half, I seem to be getting younger. If this were simply my own personal experience, I certainly wouldn't presume to write about it, or try to tell others how to achieve it. The amazing thing is that I am not alone. In fact, I seem to be surrounded by people having similar experiences. Movie stars like Raquel Welch and Jane Fonda are proudly publicizing their chronological age while visually defying it. Even the media are touting increased longevity . . . it's the hottest topic in magazines every month. Advertisements now use older, more natural looking models to sell more than just laxatives. There seems to be a growing awareness that people can remain vibrant, healthy, and attractive well into their later years. And the key ingredient, I believe, is more than exercise and good diet. It is love.

Case #1: David is 48 at the time of this writing. We met and fell in love one and a half years ago. In that time, he has "youthed" at least 10 years, maybe more. His explanation: being in love; using Zia Cosmetics; and a change of lifestyle that includes yoga classes, long walks on the beach, and extended periods of stress-free time in the mountains.

Case #2: Lillian is 84 years old and lives alone in Florida. Her second husband died 7 years ago. She has a daughter who lives 3,000 miles away and visits 2 to 3 times a year. Her only son, a Vietnam veteran, lives in seclusion, avoiding contact with all family members. Four months ago Lillian suffered a heart attack two days after returning from a cruise to Alaska. The doctor told her that had she not been in such excellent physical condition, she would not have survived.

All things considered, Lillian could be a lonely woman with no reason to get out of bed each day. But this is not the case. Lillian begins each day with a 30 minute swim in her pool. Prior to the heart attack she followed the swim with a brisk walk and a round of golf. Now she does a little yoga (that she has practiced for 25 years).

Each summer Lillian goes to Central Washington University in Washington state where she takes 4- to 5-month-long courses in such subjects as astronomy, modern history, and sign language for chimpanzees. Lillian's love is learning. "It's important to keep your mind alert and to have a hobby." A former grade school teacher, Lillian's other love is children. Once a week she volunteers as an assistant in a local kindergarten. She also works 1 day a week teaching math and reading to third and fifth grade students with learning disabilities. Last summer, after taking a summer course in the writing of family histories, Lillian bought a new typewriter and began to write her memories. This morning she told me, "I have a lot of living to do."

Case #3: Jackie is fiftysomething and very attractive. She was in good shape, dressed beautifully, and always looked great. She exercised every morning and ran her own interior decorating business. After being divorced for 12 years, she had convinced herself that she was perfectly happy being single. She didn't need a man's financial support, and she did all of the things she enjoyed, either by herself or with friends. To me, she seemed perfectly happy and led a terrific life. But Jackie felt that something was missing so she attended a seminar on relationships; that brought up some issues of which she had not been aware. Two weeks after the seminar ended, she met her "soul mate." And a few months after that, I saw a physical change in her that I could hardly believe. She looked younger, prettier, more alive and vibrant than I'd ever seen her. She also became more relaxed. And this was a woman who was terrific to begin with . . . she got even better!

Betty Friedan, author of *The Fountain of Age* (Simon and Schuster), says, "I did an enormous amount of research that shows that the definition of age—deterioration, decline, Alzheimer's, and senility—is not true. I found from my research that what happens to you after 50, after the reproductive years, more than any other period of your life, depends on what you choose to do. It isn't programmed biologically. To have purpose is essential for vital age. Bonds of intimacy are crucial for vital age. I'm talking about the kind of intimacy of which the sexual act is only one expression."

Bonnie Siegler, West Coast editor of *Longevity* magazine, writes that actress Jane Seymour had a near-death experience five years ago, the result of an allergic reaction to an injection of antibiotics. "I had an out-of-body experience, which I had never believed in. It was the white light, the whole thing." When she recovered, she was left with the realization that "the only thing that really mattered was loving somebody and being loved." She says that she "refused to die," because of her love for her two children. But she now believes that "loving someone else" is the key to her excellent health and good looks. "I feel happier when I am in a relationship or being loved. I take better care of myself and I am healthier. When I'm not in a relationship, I become depressed and put myself under a lot of stress. Then my health falters. If you are happy and involved in living life to the fullest, more open and giving, then all the energies come into place and the whole package works."

It should seem apparent by now that the journey toward "falling in love" begins with self. That was the path that so many of us chose to take in the sixties. The natural progression began with turning our gaze inward, forgiving ourselves for who we weren't, accepting who we were, and finding our place in the cosmic scheme of things. We were then able to direct our focus outside of ourselves, and suddenly we became aware of a whole world full of people who needed our love and attention. We traveled, joined the Peace Corps, and became expatriates as others in an earlier, idealistic generation had. Inspired or disillusioned, we took jobs and began careers, giving all of our creative attention and energy to "making something of ourselves" and building our careers. At some point after that, most of us met a "significant other" and focused our love on that particular individual. Then many of us started families. Suddenly we had a new kind of relationship—parenthood—and a new focus for our love—children. The children grew and we grew up with them. By the time they were on their own, we had begun to relax into a sense of who we really were.

It was at that point that many of us noticed that our priorities were changing. It seemed we'd come full circle and that it was time to get back in touch with our spiritual selves. Some of us joined churches or New Age spiritual groups; others began their journey by reading some of the books that addressed this subject, often ones that happened to be on the *New York Times* Best-seller List (always a good indication of the pulse of the times) such as Marianne Williamson's *Return to Love*, James Redfield's *The Celestine Prophecy*, and Shakti Gawain's *Return to the Garden*. Now that mainstream America has obviously entered the same path, according to the aforementioned best-seller list, we're realizing that there is more to life than earning a living, raising a family, or what we're going to eat and wear tomorrow. Quality of life has taken an upward turn, not in dollars, but in awareness. If we're going to live longer, we want to feel and look as good as possible. Now that people are beginning to take a real interest in their own well-being, they're also taking responsibility for that well-being. Now that we know how to eat and exercise properly, we can focus on how to be happy! I believe that finding love in every corner of your life is the best (and easiest) way to be truly happy.

Think of all the songs written about love—"Love Makes the World Go Round," "Love Is All There Is," "Love Is a Many Splendored Thing," "I Can't Give You Anything but Love, Baby," "Love Is a Wonderful Thing," "Money Can't Buy You Love," "Love Will Find a Way," "Love Walked In," "Love's Got a Hold on Me," and "Lovin' Her Was Easier than Anything I'll Ever Do Again"—to name just a few.

Love can even inspire a person with no literary aspirations, who has never written a poem before in his life, to write this:

> Love is a feeling like no other
> It heightens my senses
> I laugh harder
> I cry easier
> I smile wider
> I breathe deeper
> Love is a blessing
> My lover is my gift
>
> David Charnack, 1994

Regardless of how old you are, how in or out of shape, rich or poor, serious or silly, highly educated or street-smart, "There's someone for everyone" and "All you need is love."

Recommended Reading and Resources

I hope that this book has piqued your interest in many ways, and I encourage you to broaden your scope of knowledge by learning more about diverse areas of health and beauty, mind and body. I have listed below some books I recommend for gaining further information about the topics I have addressed.

Books about the Aging Process and the Mind–Body Connection

Ageless Body, Timeless Mind: The Quantum Alternative to Growing Old, Deepak Chopra, M.D. (Harmony Books, 1993)

Aging and the Skin, Dr. Albert Kligman (Raven, 1989)

Growing Younger, Dr. Robert F. Morgan with Jane Wilson (Stein and Day, 1983)

In Pursuit of Youth, Betty and Si Kamen (Dodd Mead, 1984)

Life Extension: A Practical Scientific Approach, Durk Pearson and Sandy Shaw (Warner Books, 1987)

The Life Extension Revolution, Saul Kent (Morrow, 1980)

Books about Menopause

The Change: Women, Aging and the Menopause, Germaine Greer (Fawcett-Columbine, 1991)

Hormones: The Woman's Answerbook, Louis Jovanovic, M.D., and G. Suback-Sharpe (Fawcett-Columbine, 1987)

Is It Hot in Here or Is It Me? Gayle Sand (Harper Perennial, 1993, 1994)

Menopause: A Guide for Women and Those Who Love Them, Winnifred B. Cutler, Ph.D., and Ramon Garcia, M.D. (W. W. Norton & Company, 1992)

Menopause Naturally, Sadja Greenwood, M.D. (Volcano Press, 1992)

Menopause and Osteoporosis, Linda Rector-Page (Healthy Healing Publications, Inc., 1993)

Menopause Without Medicine, Linda Ojeda (Hunter House, 1989)

The Pause: Positive Approaches to Menopause, Lonnie Barbach (Dutton, 1993)

Menopause—A Second Spring: Making A Smooth Transition With Traditional Chinese Medicine, Honora Wolfe (Blue Poppy Press, 1990)

Without Estrogen: Natural Remedies for Menopause and Beyond, Dee Ho (Carol Southern Books, 1994)

Books about Nutrition and Supplements

The Complete Guide to Anti-Aging Nutrients, Sheldon Hendler, M.D., Ph.D. (Simon and Schuster, 1985)

Diet For A Small Planet, Frances Moore Lappé (Ballantine, 1991)

Fit For Life, Harvey Diamond and Marilyn Diamond (Warner Books, 1987)

The Life Extension Weight Loss Program, Durk Pearson and Sandy Shaw (Doubleday, 1987)

Mega-Nutrition, Richard A. Kunin, M.D. (Plume, 1981)

Nutrition Against Aging, Michael A. Weiner, Ph.D., and Kathleen Goss (Bantam Books, 1983)

The Practical Encyclopedia of Natural Healing, Mark Bricklin (Fine Communications, 1994)

Sugar Blues, William Dufty (Warner Books, 1993)

Books about Herbs and Amino Acids

Detoxification and Body Cleansing, Linda Rector-Page (Healthy Healing Publications, Inc., 1993)

Fighting Infections With Herbs, Linda Rector-Page (Healthy Healing Publications, Inc., 1993)

Healthy Healing, Linda Rector-Page (Healthy Healing Publications, Inc., 1990)

Renewing Female Balance, Linda Rector-Page (Healthy Healing Publications, Inc., 1993)

Books and Videotapes about Callanetics

Write to Callanetics, 1700 Broadway, Suite 200, Denver, CO 80290; or phone 800-8-CALLAN, ext. 93.

Books and Videotapes about Yoga

Golden Yoga: Breathing, Stretching, Meditation for Seniors, Ravi Singh

Yoga Journal magazines

Yoga Practice for Beginners, Patricia Walden (800-722-7347)

Books about Aromatherapy

Aromantics, Valerie Worwood (Pan Books, 1987)

Aromatherapy for Women, Maggie Tisserand (Healing Arts Press, 1988)

Aromatherapy An A to Z, Patricia Davis (C. W. Daniel, 1988)

The Art of Aromatherapy, Robert Tisserand (Healing Arts Press, 1977)

The Aromatherapy Book, Jeanne Rose (North Atlantic Books, 1992)

The Complete Book of Essential Oils and Aromatherapy, Valerie Ann Worwood (New World Library, 1991)

Handbook of Aromatherapy, Marcel F. Lavabre (Marcel Lavabre, 1986)

Practical Aromatherapy, Shirley Price (Thorsons Publishing Group, 1987)

Practice of Aromatherapy, Jean Valnet (Destiny Books, 1980)

Scentual Touch, Judith Jackson (Henry Holt, 1986)

Books about Cellulite

The Cellulite Solution, Laura Simms (Natural Press, 1990)

Other Books by Zia Wesley-Hosford

Being Beautiful (Whatever Press, 1983)

Putting On Your Face (Bantam Books, 1985)
Face Value (Bantam Books, 1986)
Skin Care For Men Only (Harcourt, Brace, Jovanovich, 1987)
The Beautiful Body Book (Bantam Books, 1989)
Face Value: The Revised Edition (Zia Cosmetics, 1990)

Glossary of Cosmetic Terms

Abrasive: A grainy or powdered substance usually from mineral or synthetic sources. Used in cosmetics as an exfoliant to remove dead skin cells. Can be irritating and may cause small tears on skin surface.

Acetylated: Any organic compound that has been heated with acetic anhydride or acetyl chloride to remove its water. Acetylated lanolins are used in hand creams and lotions. Acetic anhydride produces irritation and necrosis of tissues in vapor state and carries a warning against contact with skin and eyes.

Acid: Substances that comprise the lower end of the pH scale, from 0 to 7, are considered to be acid in nature. Citric acid is an example of an acid substance commonly used in cosmetics. The skin has a pH of between 4.5 and 5.5; this is what is meant by "acid balance" of the skin. Since all soaps or synthetic detergents will disturb the skin's natural pH balance, it is important either to use a balanced cleansing product or to follow cleansing with a pH balanced (acid balanced) toner. Products that are highly acidic can irritate or burn the skin.

Alkali: The term originally covered the caustic and mild forms of potash and soda; now a substance is regarded as an alkali if it gives hydroxyl ions in solution. An alkaline aqueous solution is one with a pH greater than 7. Sodium bicarbonate is an example of an alkali that is used to neutralize excess acidity in cosmetics.

Alkaline: Substances that comprise the upper end of the pH scale, from 7 to 14, are considered to be alkaline in nature. Baking soda is an example of an alkaline substance. In order for soaps or detergents to work, they must be alkaline.

Allergen: Any substance that causes a reaction through skin absorption, inhalation, or ingestion. The most common allergen in cosmetics is fragrance.

Alphahydroxy acids: A group of naturally occurring acids. The sources of these acids include certain fruits (grapes, citrus, apples) as well as sour milk (lactic acid), sugarcane (glycolic acid), and red wine (tartaric acid). These acids work by loosening the protein bonds that hold the outermost layer of skin together, allowing dead skin cells to slough off. They also assist in the formation of new skin cells.

Antioxidant: A substance that inhibits the oxidation or breakdown of an ingredient or formulation. When oxidation occurs, oils turn rancid and cosmetics spoil. Vitamin E is a natural antioxidant.

Antiseptic: Germ killer.

Astringent: An ingredient that has a tightening and antiseptic effect on the skin; can be drying to the skin if used on a daily basis. Most astringent cosmetic formulations contain a base of alcohol and/or witch hazel. Aloe vera is a natural astringent that is commonly used in cosmetics.

Botanical infusion: Plants, herbs, or flowers soaked in water to form a "tea." This process is especially useful with plants that are rich in aromatic oils.

Buffering agent: An ingredient used to maintain the pH level of a cosmetic product.

Cellular renewal: The continual process of cell replacement in the skin. It takes approximately 28 days for a cell to be born and to make the journey from the bottom-most layer of skin to the surface. By the time a cell reaches the skin's surface, it has lost most of its water content and appears dry and thin. The "old cells" that reach the surface fall off by themselves or are sloughed off during the process of cleansing or exfoliating. The entire process of birth, death, and sloughing off slows down as a result of age, ultraviolet light exposure, and impaired bodily function caused by sickness, improper nutrition, drugs, etc.

Chemicals: A combination of molecules found in everything except light and electricity. Both natural and synthetic ingredients are composed of chemicals.

Comedogenic: Any topically applied cosmetic product or ingredient that can cause the formation of comedones (acne, pimples, blackheads), such as irritating chemicals, occlusive creams, or certain oily ingredients that attract or hold impurities onto the skin.

Cream: A combination of water and oil held together by an emulsifying agent.

CTFA: Cosmetics, Toiletry and Fragrance Association, a private industry organization whose purpose is self-regulation of the cosmetics industry. The CTFA Cosmetic Ingredient Dictionary is the primary source for the nationally accepted names of cosmetic ingredients.

D&C colors: Synthetic colors certified by the FDA for use in drugs and cosmetics. Colors are divided into two classifications: those "subject to certification" and those "exempt from certification." The former includes colors that may contain coal tar dyes (whose safety is subject to evaluation), while the latter includes colors of natural origin such as iron oxides and titanium dioxide.

Dermatologist-tested: This indicates that the product has been tested for safety by one dermatologist. It does not necessarily indicate that the product is completely safe, effective, or hypoallergenic.

Detergent: Any of a group of synthetic, organic, liquid, or water-soluble cleansing agents that, unlike soap, are not prepared from fats and oils and are not inactivated by hard water. Most of them are made from petroleum derivatives but vary widely in composition; some are derived from coconut oil. The major advantage of detergents is that they do not leave a hard-water scum; they also have wetting agent and emulsifying properties. Toxicity of detergents depends upon alkalinity. Dishwasher detergents, for instance, can be dangerously alkaline, whereas detergents used in cosmetic products have an acidity–alkalinity ratio near that of normal skin.

Dispersing agent: An ingredient that helps another ingredient remain suspended in a liquid, gas, or solid phase. Xanthan gum is a natural and commonly used cosmetic dispersing agent.

Emollient: A substance that has a softening effect on the skin. Vegetable oils, lanolin oil, and cetyl alcohol are natural emollients commonly used in cosmetics.

Emulsifier: An ingredient that helps to bind oil and water together into a creamy form. Egg yolk and lecithin are natural emulsifiers.

Emulsion: What is formed when two or more nonmixable liquids are shaken so thoroughly together that the mixture appears to be homogenized. Most oils form emulsions with water.

Enzyme: A protein formed in plant and animal cells or made synthetically that acts as a catalyst in chemical reactions.

Essential oil: Not oil but a volatile fluid contained within plants that carries the odor characteristic of the plant. Usually derived by a physical process such as distillation. The complex composition of individual oils makes it impossible to duplicate them synthetically. Essential oils serve as the plant's immune system.

Ester: A chemical compound formed by reacting an acid with an alcohol. Esters are used in many types of cosmetics such as lotions, moisturizers, shampoos, and cleansers. Some common esters are carbonates, from carbonic acid; laurates, from lauric acid (derived from coconut fatty acid); stearates, from stearic acid (tallow or vegetable sources); and acetates, from acetic acid.

Exfoliant: Any ingredient or product whose purpose is to remove dead skin cells from the skin's surface. Can be in the form of abrasives (facial scrubs) or nonabrasives (enzyme or chemical peels).

Extract: A liquid material prepared by distillation of a plant in alcohol. Extracts are less concentrated than essential oils but more concentrated than the plant material itself.

Fatty acids: Natural acids such as linoleic, linolenic, oleic, and stearic, that occur in varying amounts in all natural oils. These are beneficial to the skin when used both internally and externally; they help to keep it moist and to prevent dryness.

FD&C colors: Synthetic colors certified by the FDA for use in food, drugs, and cosmetics. Colors are divided into two classifications: those "subject to certification" and those "exempt from certification." The former includes colors that may contain coal tar dyes (whose safety is subject to evaluation), while the latter includes colors of natural origin such as iron oxides and titanium dioxide.

Fragrance: A wide range of synthetic chemicals or essential oils that impart a scent. Essential oils in cosmetics are usually listed by name, whereas a synthetic fragrance (often with numerous components) can be listed simply as "fragrance." Synthetic fragrances can potentially be allergens.

Humectant: An ingredient that attracts and holds moisture. In a cosmetic formulation, the humectant attracts moisture (water) from either the formulation or the air and holds it onto the skin. However, if neither the formulation nor the air contain sufficient water, the humectant will draw moisture from the skin itself. For this reason, it is important that cosmetic formulations contain sufficient amounts of water and do not contain more than 20 percent humectants.

Hydrolyzed protein: A natural protein made water-soluble by reacting the protein with an enzyme, acid, or other substance. Sources for cosmetics use can be either animal or vegetable.

Hypoallergenic: "Hypo" means "less," so "hypoallergenic" means less likely to cause allergic reaction.

Laked colors: Organic pigments used widely in cosmetics. Produced by combining an organic dye and an absorbent mineral such as iron, calcium, copper, or aluminum.

Liposome: A microscopic-sized globule of lipids (fats) and protein whose configuration resembles that of a human skin-cell membrane. Has the ability to penetrate deeply into the skin to "seek out" a lipid-poor (dry) area where it "melts" over a period of 10 to 12 hours, depositing its lipid-rich contents. Originally used by the medical industry to carry medications into the skin; now used in cosmetics as a transport system.

Lubricant: Same as emollient.

Natural: Occurring in nature; can be animal, vegetable, or mineral. There is currently no standard for the term "natural" in cosmetics.

Nonionic: A group of emulsifiers used in hand creams. They resist freezing and shrinkage.

Occlusive: Any ingredient that "seals" the skin by forming a physical barrier. Occlusives can protect the skin from the harsh effects of wind and cold, but they can also be comedogenic, clogging pores and preventing the release of toxins. They can inhibit the skin's respiration and prohibit the evaporation of water from the surface.

pH (potential hydrogen): The scale used to measure the acidity or alkalinity of solutions, ranging from 0 (indicating acidity) to 14 (indicating alkalinity). The skin has an acid balance of 4.5 to 5.5. The pH of pure water is 7, which is considered neutral.

Photosensitivity: A condition in which the application or ingestion of certain chemicals (such as propylparaben) causes skin problems, including rash, hyperpigmentation, or swelling, when the skin is exposed to sunlight.

Sensitizer: A substance that causes a reaction such as redness, itching, or swelling of the skin.

Sequestering agent: A preservative that prevents physical or chemical changes that affect the color, flavor, texture, or appearance of a product. One example is EDTA, which prevents adverse effects of metals on shampoos.

Soap: The combination of a caustic alkali (usually sodium hydroxide) and a fat or oil (tallow, coconut oil). Soaps are alkaline in composition (over 7 on the pH scale), and can be irritating to the skin. Because the FDA does not regard soap as a cosmetic, manufacturers are not required to list its ingredients on a package.

Solvent: An ingredient that helps to "solubilize" or break up a solid or nonsoluble ingredient so that it can blend into a formulation. Solvents are commonly used to help solubilize oils into water for formulations such as perfumes or bath oils.

SPF (sun protection factor): A rating system developed for sun protection products that allows the user to determine how long it is safe to stay in the sun without burning. For example, a sunscreen product with an SPF 15 allows the user to remain in the sun 15 times longer than with no protection, before burning. The SPF rating is relative to each individual's tolerance for the sun; also, this rating system only reflects protection from UVB rays, not UVA.

Stabilizer: A substance added to a product to give it body and to maintain a desired texture—for instance, the stabilizer alginic acid, which is often added to cosmetics.

Sunscreen: Sunscreen agents are the active ingredients used in over-the-counter (OTC) sunscreen products to protect against the harmful effects of UV light. This includes both UVB rays (which cause burning) and UVA rays (which contribute to photoaging and skin cancers). The FDA defines a sunscreen as an ingredient that absorbs at least 85 percent of the light in the UVB range (at wavelengths from 290 to 320 nanometers).

Surfactant: A compound that makes it easier to effect contact between two surfaces (in cosmetics, usually between the skin and a cream or lotion) by reducing surface tension. Lecithin is one example.

Synthetic: A man-made ingredient that duplicates a natural substance, or one that is unique and not found in nature. Most synthetic cosmetic ingredients are derived from petroleum.

Water (H_2O): The most common cosmetic ingredient and one whose use is standardized. Water in cosmetics must be sterilized, purified and/or filtered, demineralized, and deionized.

Wetting agent: Any of numerous water-soluble agents that promote spreading of a liquid onto a surface or penetration into a material such as skin. A wetting agent lowers surface tension for better contact and absorption.

Cosmetic Ingredient Dictionary

Albumen: Egg white. A source of pure protein. It has a soothing and tightening effect on the skin.

Algae extract: Rich in the same vital nutrients, trace elements, and amino acids present in human blood plasma, allowing it to penetrate the skin more thoroughly than most other ingredients. It speeds the elimination of toxins from cells and is a natural cellular renewal ingredient. It also helps to nourish and remineralize the skin.

Algin: A gelatinous substance derived from seaweed. It acts as an emulsifier and thickening agent.

Allantoin: A compound that occurs naturally in wheat sprouts, tobacco seed, comfrey, and sugar beets, or it may be derived synthetically from uric acid. It is an effective healing agent that helps to promote cellular renewal, and it has a soothing and softening effect on the skin.

Almond oil: A nut oil high in fatty acids. Nearly colorless and odorless, almond oil is used in soaps, moisturizers, and creams.

Aloe vera gel: A concentrated form derived from the aloe vera (true aloe) plant, one of the oldest medicinal plants known. Widely revered and used by the ancient Egyptians and Native Americans, it has remarkable healing abilities because it is a natural oxygenator (drawing and holding oxygen to the skin). For this same reason, it is one of the most effective cellular renewal ingredients available for use in cosmetics. It has a composition similar to that of human blood plasma and sea water, and because its pH is the same as human skin, it is extremely soothing and protective. It is also a natural astringent.

Annatto: A naturally occurring red-yellow dye derived from the seeds of tropical trees.

Apple cider vinegar: Found in toners; may be used with water as an "acid rinse" to adjust the skin's own pH.

Arnica extract: Used as an anti-irritant and to treat muscle soreness and bruising.

Asbestos: A proven carcinogen sometimes found in talc.

Ascorbic acid: Vitamin C. An antioxidant that is also used as a pH adjuster and as a preservative in cosmetics.

Ascorbyl palmitate: An ester of ascorbic acid. An antioxidant for oils and fats; keeps products fresh and prevents color change. *See* Ascorbic acid.

Avocado oil: Natural oil from avocados that is rich in vitamins and minerals. An excellent skin conditioner and moisturizer that readily penetrates the skin; nonocclusive.

Azulene: An essential oil derived from German camomile (*Matricaria chamomilla*). It is an excellent anti-inflammatory, analgesic, and detoxifier. Extremely calming and soothing to the skin.

Basil oil: *Ocimum basilicum* belongs to the labiate botanical family, which contains the largest number of medicinal plants. This essential oil contains linalol, thymol, tannins, pinene, and camphor, making it excellent for healing and soothing the skin. It has a stimulating effect on the skin's circulation and the oil glands, and is also balancing.

Beeswax: Natural wax produced by bees. Used in a wide variety of cosmetics as an emulsifier. Can clog pores if used as a primary ingredient in a formulation.

Bentonite: A naturally occurring clay from volcanic ash. Used as an ingredient in masks and foundation makeup.

Benzaldehyde: Artificial essential oil of almond.

Benzoic acid: Naturally occurring cosmetic preservative from gum benzoin. May be irritating to eyes. *See* Gum benzoin.

Benzophenone: UVA blocker. Protects against ultraviolet light (from sunlight and fluorescent sources).

Beta-carotene: *See* Carotene.

BHA (butylated hydroxyanisole): A synthetic antioxidant used to prevent oxidation of oils in cosmetics. Some reports of allergic reaction.

BHT (butylated hydroxythaluene): A synthetic antioxidant used to prevent oxidation of oils in cosmetics. Some reports of allergic reaction.

Bismuth oxychloride: A salt derived from the mineral bismuth that imparts a slight sheen, enabling powders to reflect light. A natural antiseptic.

Bladderwrack extract (seaweed): Derived from the dried thallus (bulbous root) of *Fucus vesiculosus,* a type of seaweed. It is rich in the same trace minerals, amino acids, and other vital nutrients present in human blood plasma and therefore helps to balance and remineralize the skin.

Bromelain: An enzyme derived from pineapples. Digests dead protein, as in surface skin cells.

2-Bromo-2-nitropropane-1, 3-diol: Can form carcinogens in cosmetics or on the skin. Often used in shampoos and moisturizers; avoid products with this ingredient. Sometimes called BNPD.

Butylene glycol: A humectant and solvent with some mold-inhibiting ability. Can be irritating if used as more than five percent of a formulation.

Butylparaben: Preservative used to prevent mold, fungus, and bacteria; extends shelf life of cosmetics. Nontoxic and nonirritating at .05 of 1 percent. (It may be irritating to the skin if more than 5 percent is used in a formulation.)

C12-15 alcohols benzoate: An emollient derived from benzoic acid, a naturally occurring preservative. Very mild.

Cajeput oil: Distilled from the flowers and leaves of the *Melaleuca leucadendra* tree, which grows in Malaysia. Antiseptic and antiviral, its function is to cleanse and drain toxins and excess oil from the skin.

Calcium carbonate (chalk): Fine white powder occurring naturally in limestone, oyster shells, and marble. Used in powders and toothpastes. Also used as an antacid, opacifier, whitener, neutralizer, filler.

Calcium silicate: Anticaking and opacifying agent; absorbent. Used in face powders, blushers, and bath salts.

Calendula: Marigold. Topical anti-inflammatory, antioxidant. Commonly used to treat acne and problem skin.

Camomile oil: Distilled from the small yellow flowers of several varieties of camomile, including German *(Matricaria chamomilla)* and Roman *(Anthemis nobilis)*. German camomile contains a high percentage of azulene, a powerful healer that is extremely soothing to the skin. In aromatherapy, camomile is used to balance female energy and reproductive organs.

Camphor: Distilled from the wood of the camphor tree *(cinnamomum camphora)*. It is a natural antiseptic and analgesic that helps to calm the skin and reduce redness.

Candelilla wax: A hard wax obtained from the candelilla plant, used as an occlusive and binder in lipsticks and creams.

Caprylic acid: Fatty acid used as an emulsifier. Found in milk and sweat and synthesized from coconut oil.

Caprylic/capric triglyceride: Barrier agent, emollient, and solvent used in foundations, eye shadow, creams, and lotions. Oily liquid from plants, vegetable oils, dairy fats, and sweat. Synthesized from coconut oil or palm kernel oil.

Carbomer: Gelling agent. Synthetic polymer used to thicken, stabilize, and promote shelf life of cosmetics. Can be irritating.

Carmine: A natural pigment derived from the dried female insect, *Coccus cacti*; used as dye.

Carnauba wax: From the Brazilian wax palm. Used as a barrier agent and texturizer in lipsticks, deodorant sticks, and depilatories.

Carotene (beta-carotene): Present in quantity in a variety of orange/yellow fruits and vegetables, such as carrots, cantaloupe, and papaya. Carotene has an orange color that oxidizes (fades) when exposed to sunlight. It is converted into vitamin A by the body, and is used for its cellular renewal and healing abilities.

Carrageenan: Sometimes called "red algae," it is derived from the type of seaweed known as "Irish moss." It is a natural emulsifier and thickening agent and has a soothing effect on the skin.

Carrot oil: Natural extract of carrot used as a colorant. High in beta-carotene; healing and soothing to the skin.

Castor oil: From the castor bean. Acts as a barrier agent, emollient, and lubricant. Used in lipsticks and moisturizers.

Cedarwood oil: From red cedar. It is a strong antiseptic and has a calming effect on the skin.

Cellulose gum: Gum from cellulose, the cell wall and structural component of plants. Used as a thickener and emulsifier in creams and lotions and as a film former in lipsticks.

Ceresin wax: From ozokerite, a naturally occurring mineral wax. Used as an emulsifier, hair conditioner, and thickener.

Ceteareth-20: A compound made from stearyl alcohol (solid alcohols mixed with stearol, a derivative of stearic acid) and coconut or palm oil. Used as an emollient and emulsifier.

Cetearyl alcohol: Not an "alcohol" such as ethyl or rubbing alcohol. It is an emulsifying wax made by combining fatty alcohols derived from vegetable sources. Used as an emulsifier and emollient, it is not drying to the skin.

Cetyl alcohol: Not an "alcohol" such as ethyl or rubbing alcohol. Yellowish white flakes with no odor or toxicity, it is used as an emollient and emulsifier. When sebum (the moisturizer produced by the body) is synthetically formulated in a laboratory, cetyl alcohol is added as one of the constituents because it closely resembles a component of sebum.

Cetyl lactate: An emollient.

Cetyl palmitate: Synthetic spermaceti.

Chlorophyll: The green component of plants used as a natural colorant in deodorants, creams, and toothpaste.

Cholesterol: Found in all body tissues. Acts as an emulsifying and lubricating agent in cosmetics.

Chondroitin sulfate: A factor of the hyaluronic acid complex that is bio-engineered (grown in a yeastlike culture in a laboratory).

Chromium hydroxide green: A coloring agent.

Citric acid: Found widely in plants and in animal tissues. Adjusts pH and acts as an antioxidant.

Citronella: An herb most commonly used as an insect repellant. In skin care, the essential oil is used to calm sebaceous glands.

Citrus oil extract: A combination of grapefruit, orange, and lemon oils.

Cocamide DEA: Acts as a foam stabilizer and thickener in shampoos.

Cocamide MEA: Appears most often in shampoos; can be mildly irritating.

Cocoa butter: A saturated fat with emollient properties, making it too heavy for use on facial skin. Frequently appears in suntan preparations. May produce contact sensitivities.

Coconut oil: A saturated fat. The fat molecules are large, making the oil too "heavy" for use on facial skin.

Collagen: The protein that makes up the fibrous support system from which skin is made. For cosmetic use, collagen is usually derived from cows. New technology has produced collagen from soy and wheat.

Colloidal sulfur: Sulfur is a naturally occurring material. Colloidal sulfur is a mixture of sulfur and acacia, a hydrophilic (water-loving) colloid derived from the African acacia tree. This ingredient is used for its ability to calm the skin and oil glands. Commonly found in various types of acne preparations, it helps to reduce redness, soreness, and swelling.

Cornflower extract: Extracted from the common flower, bachelor's button *(Centaurea cyanus)*. It contains allantoin, potassium, calcium, and vitamins C and K. Because of its soothing and anti-inflammatory properties, it is traditionally used for compresses around the eyes.

Cornstarch: A "starchy" white powder derived from corn that is very soothing to the skin. If you have an allergy to corn, you may be allergic to this ingredient.

Cucumber extract: Cucumber is a natural anti-inflammatory and has an extremely soothing effect on the skin.

Cypress oil: Possibly the most sacred, ancient essential oil, it was widely used in religious ceremonies for its spiritually "opening" effect. Distilled from the bark of the cypress tree, it is a natural astringent and restorative. As a vasoconstrictor, it also helps to shrink capillaries and calm cupreous skin.

D&C colors: *See* Glossary of Cosmetic Terms.

D&C Blue No 4: Externally except eye area.

D&C Brown No 1: Externally except eye area.

D&C Green No 5: Except eye area.

D&C Green No 6: Externally except eye area.

D&C Green No 8: Externally except eye area (0.01 percent maximum).

D&C Orange No 4: Externally except eye area.

D&C Orange No 5: Externally except eye area; lip products (5 percent maximum).

D&C Orange No 10: Externally except eye area.

D&C Orange No 11: Externally except eye area.

D&C Red No 6: Except eye area.

D&C Red No 7: Except eye area.

D&C Red No 17: Externally except eye area.

D&C Red No 21: Except eye area.

D&C Red No 22: Except eye area.

D&C Red No 27: Except eye area.

D&C Red No 28: Except eye area.

D&C Red No 30: Except eye area.

D&C Red No 31: Externally except eye area.

D&C Red No 33: Externally except eye area; lip products (3 percent maximum).

D&C Red No 34: Externally except eye area.

D&C Red No 36: Externally except eye area; lip products (3 percent maximum).

D&C Violet No 2: Externally except eye area.

D&C Yellow No 7: Externally except eye area.

D&C Yellow No 8: Externally except eye area.

D&C Yellow No 10: Except eye area.

D&C Yellow No 11: Externally except eye area.

Ext. D&C Violet No. 2: Externally except eye area.

Ext. D&C Yellow No. 7: Externally except eye area.

Deionized water: "Deionization" means that all the ions of soluble salts have been removed. Calcium, magnesium, sulfur, etc., can interfere with formulations and "deactivate" active ingredients.

Dichlorobenzyl alcohol: A type of alcohol used as a preservative. Nondrying to the skin.

Dihydroxyacetone: The "tanning agent" in many self-tanning formulas. It is actually a keto sugar that reacts with protein on the surface of the skin to create the look of a tan. The molecules in this ingredient are too large to penetrate the skin any deeper than the top-most layer. Since it is unable to react in any way with the melanin in the skin, this ingredient does not afford the protection from sun that a real tan would.

Dimethicone: An oil derived from silicone (which is derived from silica, a substance that occurs naturally in rocks and sand). Dimethicone is used to facilitate smooth application of a product, and helps to soften the skin.

Dimethicone copolyol: A more waterproof form of dimethicone that adheres better to skin and hair.

Dioctyl adipate: One component of an ester blend of oils designed to effectively penetrate the skin. It is synthetically derived and nonirritating to the skin or eyes.

Disodium EDTA: Sequestering agent. *See* EDTA.

EDTA (ethylene diamine tetraacetic acid): A synthetic chemical that removes metals or mineral ions from a solution. Used as a preservative. Can be irritating to the skin if more than 5 percent is used in a formulation.

Elastin: Animal protein found in the dermal layers of skin that functions to maintain skin elasticity. When applied topically, there is no proof that this highly insoluble protein has the ability to improve the elasticity of the skin.

Ethylparaben: A preservative. *See* Parabens.

Evening primrose oil: A source of vitamin E and gamma linoleic acid. Helps to regenerate skin cells.

Farnesol: A sesquiterpene alcohol, occurring naturally in many essential oils such as camomile, rose, citronella, sandalwood, and lemon grass. Deodorant and bacteriostat.

FD&C colors: *See* Glossary of Cosmetic Terms.

FD&C Blue No. 1: Except eye area.

FD&C Green No 3: Except eye area.

FD&C Red No 4: Externally except eye area.

FD&C Red No 40: Except eye area.

FD&C Yellow No 5: Except eye area.

FD&C Yellow No 6: Except eye area.

Fluorocarbons: A component of aerosols that destroys the ozone layer of the atmosphere.

Formaldehyde: A pungent colorless gas. Used as a preservative, disinfectant, germicide, antifungal and embalming fluid. Extremely toxic and irritating to mucous membrane; carcinogenic. Commonly used in nail polish.

Fructose: Sugar found in honey and fruits. Used as flavoring and as a humectant.

Geranium oil: Distilled from the leaves of *Pelargonium graveolens*. It is a natural antiseptic and astringent that also promotes healing. Geranium has the unusual ability to balance sebum production (because it is an adrenal cortex stimulant), making it valuable for those with combination, dry, dehydrated, or oily skin. Aromatherapists use it as an antidepressant.

Glycerin: A humectant (water-attracting/binding ingredient) that occurs naturally in both vegetable oils and animal oils. The most common source is beef lard, but this type of glycerin is usually mixed with vegetable oils when used in cosmetics.

Glyceryl cocoate: Glycerin by-product of coconut oil. Emulsifier and surfactant.

Glyceryl oleate: Used as an emulsifier in lotions and creams. Contact with eyes may cause irritation.

Glyceryl stearate: An ester used as an emulsifier (to help combine oils with water). It is a clear, oily liquid readily able to penetrate the skin, made by combining glycerin and stearic acid.

Glyceryl stearate SE: Used in shampoos as a pearlizing agent, and as an emulsifier and opacifier in creams and lotions.

Glycols: Glycerin combined with alcohol—for example, propylene glycol.

Grapefruit seed extract: Extracted from grapefruit seeds and used in combination with propylene glycol and glycerin as a preservative, bactericide, and stabilizer.

Grape seed oil: Ultrafine oil expressed from grape seeds commonly used as a carrier oil in aromatherapy products and as a base for moisturizers.

Green papaya concentrate: Made from raw, green papayas at the time when the papain (proteolytic enzyme) content is at its highest. Once the fruit begins to ripen, its enzyme content decreases substantially. A low-heat extraction and concentration process must be used to protect the active enzyme. It is an excellent free-radical scavenger and cellular renewal ingredient. Papain has the ability to digest protein, and selectively digests only dead skin cells without harming the living ones.

Guaiazulene: Commonly known as azulene. This is a component of the essential oil distilled from the blossoms of the German camomile *(Matricaria chamomilla)* flowers. It is used for its soothing and calming effect on the skin, and it also has remarkable antibacterial and antiinflammatory abilities. It has a natural bluish color that changes to green as it begins to oxidize or age.

Guanine: Provides luminescence to liquid cosmetics. From fish scales, sugar beets, yeast, and clover seed.

Guar gum: Naturally occurring resin from seeds of an Asian tree. Used as a thickener and emulsifier.

Gum benzoin: Resin from benzoin. Mild natural preservative.

Hectorite: Naturally occurring clay used in facial masks to draw out oil. May also draw moisture from skin. Gelling agent and thickener.

Honey: Used as an emollient, humectant, and bacteriostat.

Horse chestnut extract: An herb used for its calming effect on the skin.

Horsetail extract: *Equisetum arvense,* commonly known as horsetail, mare's tail, shave grass, or bottle brush, is a plant that grows throughout central Europe. It is a natural astringent that is extremely high in silica, which has a softening and smoothing effect on the skin. It also helps to strengthen vein and capillary walls, and it is high in a variety of minerals including potassium, manganese, sulfur, and magnesium.

Hyaluronic acid: A protein occurring in the skin. Known as a water binder, it is able to bind 1000 times its weight in water.

Hybrid safflower oil: The polyunsaturated oil of the herb safflower, which is high in linoleic and linolenic acids. It has a small molecular structure that allows it to be quickly absorbed. Nourishing and soothing to the skin.

Hydrocotyl extract: *Hydrocotyl asiatica,* commonly known as gotu kola or Indian pennywort, is imported from India. For hundreds of years, this plant has been called "the longevity plant" because of its incredible ability to speed cellular renewal and increase longevity. Its properties are very similar to those of ginseng. Applied to the skin, it acts as an anti-inflammatory agent; it speeds cell production and therefore is healing. It has a balancing and calming effect and is extremely soothing for aggravated or problem skin.

Hydrolyzed animal protein: A by-product of the beef industry. Helps skin to hold moisture; imparts a glossy sheen to hair.

Hydroquinone: Used as a skin bleaching agent and as an antioxidant to prevent rancidity. Causes sensitivity to sunlight. Toxic if taken internally.

Hydroxypropyl methylcellulose: A natural gelatin derived from vegetable fibers; used as a thickening agent.

Imidazolidinyl urea: A preservative that may be derived from either methanol (wood alcohol) or allantoin. Kills harmful microorganisms. It is nonirritating, nontoxic, and not a formaldehyde donor. If heated to high temperatures, such as over the boiling point, it does produce formaldehyde. Not to be confused with urea from bovine sources.

Iron oxide: A naturally occurring compound of iron and oxygen found in a wide range of colors from black to yellow. Used as a natural colorant.

Isopropyl alcohol: Dissolves oils; has antiseptic properties. Can be drying to the skin if used as a primary ingredient in a formulation.

Isopropyl lanolate: An emollient that acts as a wetting agent for cosmetic pigments. Appears as a binder for pressed powders and as a lubricant in lipsticks.

Isopropyl myristate: Used as an emollient and lubricant in preshaves, aftershaves, shampoos, bath oils, antiperspirants, deodorants, and various creams and lotions. More than 5 percent in a formulation can cause skin irritation and clog pores.

Isopropyl palmitate: Used in many moisturizing creams. It forms a thin layer on the skin and easily penetrates.

Jojoba oil: *Simondsia chinensis* is a thick, waxy oil extracted from the large, vanilla-shaped beans of a bush that grows in the arid climates of Arizona, southern California, and New Mexico. Jojoba oil is strikingly similar to human sebum and is able to effectively penetrate the skin. It is a natural cellular renewal ingredient as well as an excellent moisturizer.

Kaolin: A white Chinese clay used to give color and "slip" to powders. It also helps to gently absorb oil on the surface of the skin. Although commonly used in clay facial masks, it may be drying to the skin in this type of product.

Karite nut butter: Oil from a native African tree. Anti-irritant. Traditionally used as a sunscreen. *See* Shea butter.

Kukui oil: Oil from the Hawaiian kukui nut. Very emollient and moisturizing.

Lactic acid: One of the alphahydroxy acids; found in fermented milk. Helps to loosen "intercellular glue" holding dead skin cells onto surface of the skin. Reduces wrinkles and improves skin texture.

Laneth-10 acetate: Derived from lanolin. Acts as an emulsifier and a superfatting agent, and it has some humectant properties.

Lanolin: An oil extracted from the wool of sheep without causing any harm to the animal. It is one of the oils closest to human sebum, making it an excellent moisturizing ingredient. Lanolin is a natural emulsifier and humectant that absorbs water and holds it to the skin to help prevent dryness. Formerly believed to be a common allergen, it is now known to cause allergic reactions in only a very small percentage of people.

Lanolin alcohol: Used as a thickener for shampoos and bath gels. Gives many cosmetics a creamy texture and a high gloss.

Lanolin oil: "Dewaxed lanolin"; acts as a skin moisturizer and reduces stickiness of creams and lotions. Also found in hair conditioners, fingernail conditioners, and skin cosmetics.

Lauramide DEA: Nonionic surfactant; builds and stabilizes foam in shampoos and bubble baths. Can be drying to the skin.

Laureth-23: A nonionic surfactant found in shampoos.

Lavender oil: The most versatile of all essential oils. Because of the high percentage of linalool that it contains, lavender oil is excellent for promoting healing and for balancing the skin. It is an antiseptic, analgesic, antibiotic, antidepressant, bactericide, decongestant, and sedative. It helps to reduce scarring and also stimulates the growth of new cells.

Lecithin: A thick, oily substance present in all living cells, whether animal or plant. A natural antioxidant, emulsifier, and emollient. Also a phospholipid with great water-binding ability. (It is able to bind 300 times its weight in water.) Occurs naturally in eggs, milk, sunflower seeds, soybeans, and some vegetables.

Lemon grass oil: An essential oil distilled from the grassy herb of the same name. It is purifying, refreshing, and hydrating.

Lemon oil: An essential oil that is pressed from the outer rind of lemons. It is a mild bleach, which enables it to brighten dull skin color and calm redness. It is also a natural astringent, antiseptic, and bactericide with the ability to stimulate the white corpuscles that defend the body. The essential oil is used to regulate and control fluid accumulation and to bring balance to fluids in skin cells. Lemon also balances the pH of the skin by counteracting acidity on its surface. It has an uplifting and refreshing effect when inhaled.

Magnesium: Occurs naturally in great quantity in the sea salts from the Dead Sea, some of the most beneficial salts known. Magnesium helps to remineralize and soothe the skin.

Magnesium aluminum silicate: A naturally occurring mineral that is commonly used to emulsify, thicken, and color cosmetics. Because of its enormous molecular size, it is not absorbed through the skin.

Magnesium carbonate: Found in powders and covering preparations.

Magnesium silicate: *See* Talc.

Magnesium stearate: A compound of magnesia (a naturally occurring white alkaline powder) and stearic acid used as a natural coloring agent.

Manganese: Occurs naturally in great quantity in the sea salts from the Dead Sea, some of the most beneficial salts known. Manganese is soothing and calming to the skin.

Manganese violet: A light violet powder; can be used around the eyes.

Matricaria oil: Known as azulene. An essential oil distilled from flowers of *Matricaria chamomilla*, or German camomile. One of its major components, chamazulene, is an effective anti-inflammatory that encourages healing. Another component, bisabolol, is a powerful antiseptic and antimicrobial. This oil also contains flavonoids, plant acids, fatty acids, amino acids, polysaccharides, salicylate derivatives, choline, and tannin. Azulene is extremely soothing to the skin and has a distinctive smell, much like fresh hay. Only tiny amounts of this powerful essential oil need to be used for product effectiveness. Aromatherapists use it as an anti-inflammatory, analgesic, antidepressant, antifungal, and disinfectant. Excellent for the treatment of dry, reddened, burned, or sensitive skin.

Menthol: An antiseptic and anesthetic found in skin lotions and shave creams. Has been shown to cause adverse reactions when applied in high concentrations to the skin.

Methylparaben: A derivative of PABA (para-aminobenzoic acid). Used as a preservative with antimicrobial abilities, it prevents the formation of bacteria. Nontoxic and nonirritating at .15 of 1 percent. *Note:* This ingredient, along with butylparaben and propylparaben, may be irritating to the skin if more than 5 percent is present in a formulation; there are many commercially made cosmetics that have such a high percentage, which explains the commonly held belief that the parabens are sensitizers.

Methyl salicylate: Oil of birch, or oil of wintergreen. Anti-irritant and disinfectant. Main constituent of wintergreen oil or made synthetically. Very cooling and relaxing, but irritating to mucous membrane.

Mica: A naturally occurring silicate found in a variety of rocks. Easily distinguishable by its shape, it comes in thin, papery sheets. Mica has a natural iridescence and varies in color from brownish green and blue to colorless. It is used as a natural colorant and to impart softness to the skin.

Microcrystalline wax: Used as a stiffening and opacifying agent.

Mineral oil: A by-product of the petroleum industry. A thinner form of petrolatum (Vaseline). Contrary to its name, this is an inert substance that does not contain any minerals, nutrients, or organic ingredients. Forms an occlusive layer on the skin that "seals" it; extremely comedogenic when used as a primary ingredient in moisturizers, liquid foundation, and other cosmetics.

Montan wax: Often used in place of carnauba wax.

Mucopolysaccharides: A basic component of the skin. This gelatinous material helps maintain a moist environment for collagen, elastin, and dermal cells and provides support for connective tissue and mucous membrane. Used as a humectant and skin softener in cosmetics.

Neopentyl glycol dicaprylate/dicaprate: Used as a lubricant; soothing and softening to the skin. It is a compound of neopentyl glycol, which is derived synthetically, and dicaprylate/dicaprates, which are derived from coconut. Caprylates are in the glyceride family and are found in human sebum.

Neroli: Essential oil distilled from the flowers of the bitter orange tree. Used in aromatherapy to ease nervous tension and induce calm.

Nonoxynol-10: A synthetic ingredient used as a dispersing agent to solubilize essential oils. Not to be confused with the spermicide nonoxynol-9.

Octoxynol-1: Used as an emulsifier and dispersing agent.

Octyl methoxycinnamate: Sunscreen, UVB blocker. Derived from cinnamon or cassia oil. Less irritating than PABA.

Octyl palmitate: 2-ethylhexyl alcohol reacted with palmitic acid. *See* Palmitic acid.

Octyl stearate: The ester of 2-ethylhexyl alcohol, a fatty alcohol. Octyl stearate may be derived from tallow or vegetable oils.

Oleic acid: A common constituent of many animal and vegetable fats and, therefore, of most normal diets. Used in cosmetics as an emollient in creams and lotions. Can be mildly irritating.

Oleyl alcohol: Found in fish oils; has softening and lubricating qualities.

Olive oil: Natural oil used as an emollient in soaps, cleansers, and shampoos.

Oxybenzone: *See* Benzophenone.

Ozokerite: *See* Ceresin wax.

PABA: *See* Para-aminobenzoic acid.

Padimate-O: Brand name for PABA.

Palmarosa oil: The essential oil of palmarosa grass *(Cymbopogan martini)*. Exceptional in bringing hydration to the skin, it is also an effective cellular renewal ingredient.

Palmitate: Salt of palmitic acid. Used as an oil in many cosmetics. *See* Palmitic acid.

Palmitic acid: A natural fatty acid found in palm, cottonseed, peanut, ricebran, sorghum, and other natural vegetable oils. Used as an emulsifier, surfactant, and texturizer.

Palm kernel oil: Oil from an African palm nut. High-sudsing cleaning agent used in soaps.

Panthenol: Part of the water-soluble vitamin B complex.

Pantothenic acid: The result of a reaction in skin enzymes to panthenol. Acts as an healing agent.

Papain: An active proteolytic enzyme found in papaya; the most potent form comes from unripened green papaya. Used in exfoliants to dissolve dead skin cells.

Para-aminobenzoic acid (PABA): A sunscreening agent. Possibly phototoxic and photoallergenic; a common sensitizer.

Parabens: Broad-spectrum preservatives derived from plant or petroleum sources. Effective against bacteria, fungus, yeast, and mold. Parabens are some of the safest preservatives, effective over a wide pH scale.

Paraffin: Derived from petroleum. Used as a thickener for cosmetic creams.

PEG: An abbreviation for polyethylene glycol, a synthetic polymer used as a humectant, emulsifier, emollient, binder, solvent, and stabilizer; protects against oxidation and moisture loss. It is derived from natural gas. Higher numbers indicate more PEG chains are present in the molecule.

PEG-5 ceteth-10 phosphate: A compound of polyethylene glycol, ceteth (from coconut fruit), and ethylene oxide, with phosphoric acid (which is produced synthetically). Used as an emulsifier.

PEG-7 glyceryl cocoate: A combination of polyethylene glycol and glyceryl cocoate (derived from coconut oil) to form a type of sucrose (sugar) extract. It is a mild cleansing agent and emollient that breaks up fat on the skin's surface without stripping the skin's natural oils or causing dryness. Rinses completely from the skin with water. It may be used in place of sodium lauryl or laureth sulfate, which are both drying and stripping for the skin.

PEG-8: A polymer of ethylene oxide. Acts as an emollient, plasticizer, and softener for cosmetics creams and shampoos.

PEG-40 castor oil: A compound made from polyethylene glycol (PEG) and castor oil, an extract of the castor bean. This ingredient is used as a solvent to help disperse other ingredients in a solution.

PEG-100 stearate: Polyethylene glycol combined with stearic acid to form a water-soluble ester used as an emulsifier and emollient; has a softening effect on the skin.

Peppermint oil: An essential oil containing menthol that has a cooling effect on the skin. May be irritating to mucous membrane.

Petrolatum: Also known as petroleum jelly, paraffin jelly, Vaseline. Forms an occlusive barrier on the skin, which limits the skin's ability to function. Common comedogenic ingredient.

Phenyl mercuric acetate: Used as a preservative in shampoos and eye cosmetics. It is highly toxic if inhaled or swallowed and can cause skin irritation.

Phosphoric acid: Functions as a metal ion sequestrant and an acidifier.

Polyaminopropyl biguanide: A synthetically derived preservative. It was originally developed by Bausch and Lomb for use in eye products worn by contact lens wearers. It is one of the most gentle, yet effective, antimicrobial preservatives available.

Polysorbate 20: Derived from sorbitol. It is a water-soluble yellowish liquid used as a dispersing agent and stabilizer, and it has a soothing effect on the skin. Some allergic reactions reported.

Potassium hydroxide (caustic potash, lye): Used in the manufacture of liquid soaps and bleaches.

Potassium sodium copper chlorophyllin: A natural colorant derived from chlorophyll.

Propylene glycol: Appears in many cosmetics as a solvent, conditioning agent, and humectant. Can be irritating if more than 5 percent is used in a formulation.

Propylene glycol stearate: Functions as an emollient, thickener, and emulsion stabilizer in creams and lotions.

Propyl gallate: Acts as an antioxidant (preservative).

Propylparaben: A preservative derived from PABA that is widely used in cosmetics. Its fungicidal and antibacterial abilities help prevent yeast and mold. Nontoxic and nonirritating at .05 of 1 percent. (It may be irritating to the skin if more than 5 percent is present in a formulation.)

PVM/MA copolymer: Has thickening, dispersing, and stabilizing properties; highly irritating to eyes, skin, and mucous membrane.

PVP: Forms a hard, transparent, lustrous film. Used primarily in hair sprays.

Quaternium-15: A synthetic preservative and bactericide derived from ammonium chloride. May be irritating to the skin if more than 5 percent is used in a formulation.

Quaternium-18: Used as a conditioning agent in hair conditioners. It is an eye irritant and can cause contact dermatitis.

Quaternium-19: A substantive (clinging) hair conditioner.

Resorcinol: Irritating to the skin and mucous membrane. Sometimes used as an antidandruff agent because of its antiseptic properties.

Retinoic acid (Retin-A): Vitamin A acid. A chemical skin exfoliant. May irritate skin and cause sun sensitivity.

Retinyl palmitate: Vitamin A. A primary antioxidant vitamin, free-radical scavenger, and cellular renewal ingredient (healer).

Rice bran oil: An ingredient rich in vitamin E derived from the bran of rice. It is very similar to wheat germ oil but not as "heavy," because it has a smaller molecule that is able to more easily penetrate the skin.

Rosemary oil: An essential oil invigorating to the circulation as well as to the psyche.

Rosewood oil: Distilled from the bark of the *Aniba roseaodora* tree that grows in the Amazon rain forest. It is high in linalool, making it balancing and healing. It also has antibacterial and analgesic abilities.

Sage oil: This essential oil, like lavender, has the distinction of being either invigorating or calming, depending on what is needed at the time. Very balancing.

Salicylic acid: From benzoic acid. Used in cosmetics as a fungicide, sunscreen, and anesthetic; has a mild peeling effect. Can be irritating to the skin.

Sandalwood oil: Distilled from the heartwood of the *Santalum album* tree that grows in India. It is a very strong antiseptic as well as being extremely soothing to the skin. It also helps the skin hold water. Ayurvedic practitioners believe it to be a powerful aphrodisiac; aromatherapists use it to relieve stress and anxiety.

SD alcohol: Specially denatured ethyl alcohol, treated to become unfit for oral consumption. Used as a solvent and astringent in toners, deodorants, mouthwashes, and hairsprays. Very drying to the skin.

Shea butter: Karite nut butter. A fatty substance obtained from the nut of the karite nut tree. A natural cellular renewal ingredient, it has excellent moisturizing and nourishing abilities as well as being a natural sunblock.

Silica: A naturally occurring colorless crystal or white powder commonly found in a variety of rocks. High in various minerals, silica helps to remineralize the skin, and it also has a softening effect.

Silicone: A group of inorganic compounds of silicon and oxygen. A clear liquid used to produce slip and richness. Used as a substitute for oil in many types of products. Examples include dimethicone, dimethicone copolyol, simethicone, and cyclomethicone.

Silk powder: A by-product of the silk industry used in face powders to gently absorb excess oil that may be present on the surface of the skin.

Simethicone: A silicone oil. This clear liquid is used as an antifoaming agent, ointment base, and as a hair and skin protectant.

Sodium bicarbonate: Baking soda. Can be used to help adjust the skin's pH; extremely softening.

Sodium borate: A detergent builder, emulsifier, and preservative in cosmetics. *Caution:* ingestion of 5 to 10 grams by young children can cause severe vomiting, diarrhea, and death.

Sodium chloride: Sea salt. Remineralizes and softens the skin.

Sodium dehydroacetate: Preservative, fungicide, and bactericide.

Sodium hyaluronate: Hyaluronic acid. A cellular renewal ingredient and healing agent that is found in all human cells. Although this ingredient was originally extracted for commercial use from roosters' combs, it is now also produced synthetically.

Sodium hydroxide: Lye, caustic soda. The base alkali of soap manufacturing; also used in oven cleaners and liquid drain cleaners. Varying degrees of skin irritation.

Sodium laureth sulfate: An ionic (negatively charged) surfactant. Appropriate for use in shampoos but too stripping for use on the skin.

Sodium lauroyl sarcosinate: A mild cleansing agent derived from coconut oil. Appropriate for use in shampoos; may be too drying for use on the skin.

Sodium lauryl sulfate: Used in many cosmetics as an emulsifier and a detergent. Strongly degreases and dries the skin; okay for use in shampoo.

Sodium PCA (NaPCA): The sodium salt of pyroglutamic acid. Commonly referred to as the "natural moisturizing factor," it is found in all living cells. Its function is to help maintain the water balance in cells, which maintains the natural water balance or moisturization of the skin. The body's production of NaPCA decreases as we age.

Sorbic acid: Made from berries of the mountain ash tree. A mold inhibitor and fungicidal agent. Also acts as a humectant in cosmetic creams and lotions. Can cause redness and a slight burning sensation for some people.

Sorbitan laurate: Used as an emulsifier in many cosmetics. Found to be nonirritating to eyes and skin.

Sorbitan sesquioleate: An emulsifier; nonirritating to skin and eyes.

Sorbitan stearate: An emulsifier; non-irritating to skin and eyes.

Sorbitol: A solid, white crystalline substance very much like sugar but more than twice as sweet. It is derived from fruits such as apples, berries, cherries, pears, and plums; it may also be derived from corn syrup. It is a humectant (water-attracting/binding) ingredient as well as an emollient.

Soybean oil: A light, readily absorbed oil derived from soybeans. It is rich in fatty acids and vitamin E and has a small molecule, which allows it to easily penetrate the skin.

Spearmint oil: Derived from *Mentha spicata,* this essential oil is high in menthol, limonene, and bisabolol, as well as flavonoids, tocopherols, betaine, choline, azulene, tannin, and rosemaric acid. Milder than its cousin peppermint, it is antiseptic, antiparasitic, and anti-inflammatory. Because of the menthol it contains, it is cooling and soothing to the skin and helps to increase circulation.

Squalane: A nutrient-rich oil present in human sebum (the skin's own moisturizer) and involved in the process of cell growth. Squalane can be created synthetically or obtained from either the liver of the rare Japanese azame shark or olive oil or wheat germ oil. Squalane is also a natural bactericide and healer. It spreads evenly along the surface of the skin to coat all of its contours, nonocclusively, to protect it. Squalane is also able to penetrate deeper and more readily than most other oils. *Note:* Squalane is meant to be used topically, and should not be confused with squalene, another form of the same ingredient that has been purified for the purpose of ingestion.

Squalene: The pasteurized form of squalane. A bactericide and an emollient.

Stearalkonium chloride: Extremely effective hair conditioner and softener.

Stearic acid: One of the most common natural fatty acids, occurring in most animal and vegetable fats. It is white, waxy, thick, and unable to penetrate the skin unless combined with a substance such as glycerin. The most common sources are coconut and palm oil. When combined with PEG-100 stearate, it forms a water-soluble ingredient that is used as both an emulsifier and an emollient.

Stearyl alcohol: Pearlizing agent, lubricant, and antifoam agent.

Sucrose cocoate: A very gentle cleansing agent in the form of a sugar, derived from coconut oil. Nonstripping and nondrying to the skin, it solubilizes and washes off completely with water.

Talc (magnesium silicate): A natural mineral. Adheres to skin; used in makeup, powders and foundation; produces slip and coloring. A lung irritant when used in powder form.

TEA-lauryl sulfate: High foaming agent. Prolonged skin contact may cause skin irritation.

Tea tree oil: From the Australian tea tree, *Melaleuca alternifolia*. Germicide, fungicide, and antiseptic. This oil is commonly used for treating acne, cuts, burns, and insect bites.

Tetrasodium EDTA: Sequestering agent. Prolonged skin contact may cause irritation, possibly even a mild burn.

Thyme lemon oil: An essential oil belonging to the *medicinal labiate* family of plants; distilled from the wild-crafted herb collected in Spain. It is balancing, and it strengthens the immune system and aids cellular renewal.

Titanium dioxide: A natural white pigment that occurs in several varieties of crystal forms. It has a natural sun-blocking ability and is used to deflect ultraviolet rays and to cover flaws on the skin.

Toluene sulfonamide: Formaldehyde resin. Used as a plasticizer in nail polishes; a strong sensitizer.

Triclosan: A bactericide with very high percutaneous absorption. Can cause liver damage; an eye irritant.

Triethanolamine (TEA): An alkalizing agent in cosmetics. Can cause irritation and sensitivity if more than 5 percent is used in a formulation.

Ultramarine blue: Used as pigment.

Vetiver oil (vetivert): *Andropogon muricatus* is a scented grass similar to lemon grass and citronella that grows in India and other tropical climates. The essential oil is distilled from the root, making it the most grounding of all essential oils. It is also a very powerful humectant.

Vitamin A: "The skin vitamin"; one of three vitamins able to be absorbed by the skin (vitamins E and D are the others). It is a potent antioxidant, making it an extremely effective free-radical scavenger. It is used widely for healing and as an anti-aging ingredient because of its ability to stimulate new cell production.

Vitamin D: One of three vitamins able to be absorbed by the skin and the only one that the body is able to manufacture (when exposed to ultraviolet light). This vitamin is necessary for the building of new skin cells, as well as bones, teeth, and hair.

Vitamin E: A natural cellular renewal (healing) ingredient and antioxidant. In its pure form, the oil is too heavy for daily use on the face; however, it makes an excellent ingredient in moisturizers, eye treatment preparations, and facial masks. In its pure form, it may be used for healing cuts, abrasions, and burns.

Wheat germ glycerides: Derived by pressing wheat germ. A dietary source of vitamin E; excellent addition to moisturizers and lotions.

Wheat germ oil: Obtained from the wheat kernel. This heavy oil is used in a wide variety of cosmetic preparations. Natural source of vitamins A, E, and D, and squalane.

Witch hazel: Natural extract of the *Hamamelis* plant. Used as an astringent in cosmetics. Soothing to irritated skin; non-drying.

Xanthan gum: A thickener and emulsion stabilizer. A natural wax produced by a microorganism.

Ylang ylang oil: Extracted from the flower of the exotic ylang ylang tree, which grows in the Far East and in the tropics. This oil is a natural antiseptic, and is used in aromatherapy as a sedative, antidepressant, and aphrodisiac. It is used in cosmetics primarily as a fragrance.

Zinc: Occurs naturally in great quantity in the sea salts from the Dead Sea, some of the most beneficial salts known. Zinc helps to remineralize and calm the skin.

Zinc oxide: Widely used in powders and creams to help cosmetics adhere to the skin. A natural, physical sun-blocking ingredient.

Zinc stearate: Widely used in powders and creams to help cosmetics adhere to the skin. May be harmful if inhaled; has an effect on the lungs similar to asbestos.

Index